A Pocket B...

Inter...
Care...

Data, Drugs and Procedures

Second edition

Jack Tinker BSc FRCS FRCP DIC
Hon. Consultant Physician
The Middlesex Hospital
Postgraduate Medical Dean
University of London

Simon N. Jones MB BS MRCP (UK) FRCR
Consultant Radiologist
Poole General Hospital

Edward Arnold
A division of Hodder & Stoughton
LONDON   MELBOURNE   AUCKLAND

© 1990 Jack Tinker and Simon N. Jones

First published in Great Britain 1986

British Library Cataloguing in Publication Data

Tinker, Jack, *1936–*
  A pocket book for intensive care. — 2nd ed.
  1. Critically ill patients. Intensive care
  I. Title   II. Jones, Simon N.
  616'.028

  ISBN 0-340-51764-6

Whilst the advice and information in this book is believed to be true
and accurate at the date of going to press, neither the author nor the
publisher can accept any legal responsibility or liability for any errors
or omissions that may be made.

Typeset in 10/11pt English Times by Colset. Printed and bound in
Great Britain for Edward Arnold, the educational, academic and
medical division of Hodder and Stoughton Limited, Mill Road,
Dunton Green, Sevenoaks, Kent by Richard Clay Ltd, Bungay,
Suffolk

Preface

Second edition

Since 1986 the pocket book has been revised and expanded to incorporate changes in clinical practice and recent developments. In particular, a section on artificial ventilation and revision of parenteral feeding is included.

We are grateful for the many helpful suggestions that we have received from colleagues and reviewers. Hopefully, we have satisfied their requirements and trust that the pocket book will continue to be a success.

London 1989
JT
SNJ

Acknowledgements

We wish to thank Roger Hayward and Robert Miller for their helpful comments and Ann Knight for her valuable assistance in constructing the section on artificial ventilation. We are also grateful to Yvonne Perks for her secretarial help.

Preface

First edition

The many books about intensive care range from very large, all embracing, texts to relatively small handbooks. All of them, however, present in varying detail instruction on clinical management. This pocket book is not an addition to this range since it has been specifically compiled as a source of hopefully useful practical information for medical and nursing staff working in intensive care units or dealing with emergencies in other settings.

The contents are presented systematically, and the information given relates to physiological and technical data, drugs and their dosages, and techniques for performing important practical procedures.

We hope that this will become an established occupant of the white coat or dress pocket.

London 1986   JT
                                                                            SNJ

Contents

Haematology

Normal values for adults

Haemoglobin (Male)	13.0–17.5 g/dl
(Female)	12.0–16.0 g/dl
PCV (Male)	40–50%
(Female)	36–47%
Red cell count (Male)	$4.5–6.4 \times 10^{12}$/litre
(Female)	$3.9–5.6 \times 10^{12}$/litre
MCHC	32–36%
MCV	80–96 fl
MCH	27–32 g/dl
Reticulocyte count	0.2–2.0%
Platelet count	$150–400 \times 10^9$/litre
White cell count	
Total	$4–11 \times 10^9$/litre
Neutrophils	40–75% or 2500–7500/mm^3
	$2.5–7.5 \times 10^9$/litre
Lymphocytes	20–45% or 1500–3500/mm^3
	$1.5–3.5 \times 10^9$/litre
Monocytes	2–10% or 200–800/mm^3
	$0.2–0.8 \times 10^9$/litre
Eosinophils	1–6% or 40–440/mm^3
	$0.04–0.4 \times 10^9$/litre
Basophils	0–2% or 0–110/mm^3
	$0–0.1 \times 10^9$/litre
Sedimentation rate (Westergren)	<10 mm/hour
Serum B_{12}	140–800 ng/litre
Serum folate	2.5–20 μg/litre

Biochemistry

Normal values

Many values are affected by age, sex, time of day, fasting status, posture, diet, therapy, etc.

Blood   (Plasma or serum unless otherwise stated)

Ammonia	up to 35 μmol/litre

Bilirubin	
Total	up to 15 μmol/litre
Conjugated	< 5 μmol/litre
Caeruloplasmin	0.14–0.58 g/litre
Calcitonin	< 0.08 μg/litre
Calcium, total	2.20–2.55 mmol/litre
Chloride	91–106 mmol/litre
Cholesterol, total	4.0–7.0 mmol/litre
Complement C3	0.7–1.7 g/litre
C4	0.1–0.7 g/litre
Copper (Male)	13–23 μmol/litre
(Female)	13–26 μmol/litre
Cortisol 09.00h	140–700 nmol/litre
24.00h	less than 140 nmol/litre
Creatinine	45–110 μmol/litre
Enzymes	
Amylase	up to 300 iu/litre
Aspartate amino-transferase (AST)	up to 40 iu/litre
Creatinine kinase (CK):	
Total CK (Male)	< 270 iu/litre
(Female)	< 200 iu/litre
CK MB	< 16 iu/litre
γ Glutamyltransferase (γGT)	
(Male)	up to 60 iu/litre
(Female)	up to 30 iu/litre
α Hydroxybutyrate dehydrogenase (HBD)	up to 310 iu/litre
Phosphatase	
Acid, prostatic	up to 4 iu/litre
Alkaline (Male)	20–28 iu/litre
(Female)	20–70 iu/litre
Glucose (fasting, venous blood)	3.0–5.0 mmol/litre
Haemoglobin (plasma)	< 50 mg/litre
Haemoglobin A1 (glycosylated)	6–9%
Immunoglobulins	
IgG	5–15 g/litre
IgA	0.5–4.0 g/litre

IgM	0.5–2.0 g/litre
IgE	< 122 U/ml
Iron	15–35 μmol/litre
Iron binding capacity (TIBC)	45–70 μmol/litre
Lactate	1.0–1.8 mmol/litre
Magnesium	0.6–1.0 mmol/litre
Osmolality (plasma)	275–295 mOsmol/kg
Phosphate	0.6–1.3 mmol/litre
Potassium	3.3–4.5 mmol/litre
Proteins	
Total (plasma)	63–81 g/litre
Albumin	36–50 g/litre
Pyruvate	55–115 μmol/litre
Sodium	132–145 mmol/litre
Triglyceride	0.4–1.8 mmol/litre
Urate	0.10–0.40 mmol/litre
Urea	3.0–7.0 mmol/litre
Zinc	7–20 μmol/litre

Urine (Values per 24 hour excretion unless otherwise stated)

Calcium	2.5–7.5 mmol
Cortisol (free)	up to 400 nmol
Creatine	up to 0.4 mmol
Creatinine	9–18 mmol
Cystine	0.1–0.4 mmol
5-Hydroxyindole acetic acid (5HIAA)	up to 52 μmol
4-Hydroxy-3-methoxy-mandelic acid (HMMA)	
Normal	up to 35 μmol
Borderline	35–55 μmol
Osmolality	40–1400 mOsmol/kg
Oxalate	up to 0.4 mmol
Phosphate	15–50 mmol
Porphobilinogen	up to 45 μmol
Porphyrins	
Coproporphyrin	up to 240 nmol
Uroporphyrin	up to 30 nmol
Potassium	35–90 mmol

Protein	up to 0.15 g
Sodium	100–240 mmol
Urea	150–500 mmol
Urate	3–12 mmol

Faeces

Total moist weight	60–250 g/24 hours
Total fat (as fatty acid)	up to 5 g/24 hours
Porphyrins	
Coproporphyrin	up to 30 nmol/g dry weight
Protoporphyrin	up to 140 nmol/g dry weight

1 Cardiovascular system

Physiological data

1. Cardiovascular pressures

		Mean (mmHg)	Normal range (mmHg)
Right atrium central venous pressure (CVP)		4	0–8
Right ventricle	systolic	25	15–30
	end diastolic	4	0–8
Pulmonary artery	systolic	25	15–30
	diastolic	10	5–15
	mean	15	10–20
Pulmonary artery wedge pressure		10	5–15
Left atrium		7	4–12
Left ventricle	systolic	120	90–140
	diastolic	7	4–12
Aorta	systolic	125	90–140
	diastolic	70	60–90
	mean	85	70–105

2. Cardiac output and cardiac index

(a) Cardiac output $= \dfrac{O_2 \text{ consumption (ml/min)}}{\text{Arteriovenous } O_2 \text{ content difference (ml/litre)}}$

$\simeq 6.0$ litres/min for a 70 kg man at rest

(b) Cardiac index $= \dfrac{\text{Cardiac output (litres/min)}}{\text{Body surface area (m}^2)}$

$\simeq$ 2.2 litres/min m^{-2} for a normal 70 kg man

In 'high output' states the cardiac output can rise up to values of 25 litres/min. Figures of less than 3.0 litres/min characterize 'low output' states.

3. Mixed venous oxygen content

$$C\text{v}_{O_2} = C\text{a}_{O_2} - \dot{V}_{O_2}/\dot{Q}$$

$C\text{v}_{O_2}$ = Mixed venous oxygen content (ml/litre).
$C\text{a}_{O_2}$ = Mixed arterial oxygen content (ml/litre).
$\dot{V}_{O_2}$ = Oxygen uptake (ml/min).
$\dot{Q}$ = Cardiac output (ml/min).

$C\text{v}_{O_2}$ relates tissue oxygen delivery relative to demand. With impaired tissue oxygen delivery $C\text{v}_{O_2}$ is decreased. A reduction in mixed venous oxygen content is an indirect indicator of a falling cardiac output.

Sampling site: high right ventricle or pulmonary artery.

4. Central venous pressure (CVP)

CVP is the mean pressure in the right atrium. Its value is affected by:
  ○ Function of the right heart.
  ○ Venous tone.
  ○ Circulating blood volume.
  ○ Intrathoracic pressure.
  ○ Intrapericardial pressure.
The CVP may not be a reliable predictor of left atrial pressure.

Measurement
A catheter is inserted via either the subclavian, internal jugular or the antecubital vein so that its tip lies at the junction of the superior vena cava and right atrium.

The CVP can then be measured either intermittently with a simple fluid manometer (dextrose or saline) or continuously with a pressure transducer. The zero reference level is either at the 4th intercostal space in the midaxillary line or the manubrium sterni.

From the former the normal range is 2–8 mmHg (0.4–1.1 kPa). Normally, there is a fluctuation of value with respiration. If this fluctuation is not present, the catheter is situated peripherally, misplaced, or blocked. If a patient is ventilated by intermittent positive pressure ventilation, the mean intrathoracic pressure is increased by approximately 5 mmHg (0.7 kPa), and this is reflected by a rise in CVP.

5. Pulmonary capillary wedge pressure (PCWP)

PCWP is an indirect measurement of left atrial pressure (*see* p. 36).

6. Interpretation of changes in CVP and PCWP

CVP	PCWP	Causes
↑	Normal	Right ventricular failure
		Pulmonary embolism
		Pulmonary hypertension
		Tricuspid incompetence
↓	↓	Hypovolaemia
Normal	↑	Left ventricular failure
↑	↑	Right and left ventricular failure and hypervolaemia

7. Systemic vascular resistance

$$\text{Systemic vascular resistance (SVR)} = \frac{(MAP - MRAP) \times 80}{\dot{Q}} \text{(dyne-sec-cm}^{-5})$$

$$MAP = \frac{\text{systolic pressure} + (\text{diastolic pressure} \times 2)}{3} \text{ (mmHg)}$$

MAP = Mean arterial pressure (mmHg).
MRAP = Mean right atrial pressure (mmHg).
80 = Conversion factor.
$\dot{Q}$ = Cardiac output (litres/min).

8. Pulmonary vascular resistance

$$\text{Pulmonary vascular resistance (PVR)} = \frac{(PAM - PCWP) \times 80}{\dot{Q}} \text{(dyne-sec-cm}^{-5})$$

PAM   = Pulmonary artery mean pressure (mmHg).
PCWP = Pulmonary capillary wedge pressure (mmHg).

Practical data

1.   Intravenous infusion rates conversion table

This table shows the conversion of drops D/min (vertical
axis) into ml/hour (horizontal axis) for the common drip
counters. For example, an intravenous infusion set that
delivers 10 D/ml set at 20 D/min will infuse 120 ml/hour.

The chart has been calibrated using the 'IMED' Accudot.
It may not be true for other sets and the user is advised to
follow the particular manufacturer's instructions.

D/min	\multicolumn{6}{c}{D/ml intravenous infusion sets}					
	10	12	15	18	20	60
	ml/hour	ml/hour	ml/hour	ml/hour	ml/hour	ml/hour
1	6	5	4	3.3	3	1
2	12	10	8	6.7	6	2
3	18	15	12	10.0	9	3
4	24	20	16	13.3	12	4
5	30	25	20	16.7	15	5
6	36	30	24	20.0	18	6
7	42	35	28	23.3	21	7
8	48	40	32	26.7	24	8
9	54	45	36	30.0	27	9
10	60	50	40	33.3	30	10
15	90	75	60	50.0	45	15
20	120	100	80	66.7	60	20
25	150	125	100	83.3	75	25
30	180	150	120	100.0	90	30
35	210	175	140	116.7	105	35
40	240	200	160	133.3	120	40
45	270	225	180	150.0	135	45
50	300	250	200	166.7	150	50
55	330	275	220	183.3	165	55
60	360	300	240	200.0	180	60
65	390	325	260	216.7	195	65
70	420	350	280	233.3	210	70
75	450	375	300	250.0	225	75
80		400	320	266.7	240	80
85		425	340	283.3	255	85
90		450	360	300.0	270	90
95		475	380	316.7	285	95
99		495	396	330.0	297	99

2. Electrolyte concentrations in commonly used intravenous fluids

Solutions	Electrolyte concentration (mmol/litre)				
	Na$^+$	K$^+$	Cl$^-$	HCO$_3^-$	Ca^{2+}
Sodium chloride 0.45%	77		77		
Sodium chloride 0.9%	150		150		
Sodium chloride 5%	855		855		
Sodium bicarbonate 1.4%	167			167	
Sodium bicarbonate 2.74%	326			326	
Sodium bicarbonate 8.4%	1000			1000	
Potassium chloride 0.3% and Sodium chloride 0.9%	150	40	190		
Hartmann's solution	131	5	111	29	2
Ringer's solution	147	4	155		2
Sodium lactate (1/6 molar)	167			167	

Drugs, dosages and infusion regimens

1. Aminophylline

Use and dosage
Left ventricular failure, airways obstruction.
Intravenous bolus
    250 mg (5 mg/kg) slowly over 10–15 min.
NB
— Extreme care should be taken in patients already taking oral theophyllines. In some centres oral theophylline administration is regarded as a contraindication to systemic therapy.
— The effects of aminophylline are potentiated by cimetidine and erythromycin.
— The dose should be reduced in elderly patients and in those with impaired hepatic function.

2. Amiodarone

Uses
• Supraventricular tachycardia.
    Nodal tachycardia.
    Ventricular tachycardia.

- Atrial flutter and fibrillation.
- Treatment of dysrhythmias complicating acute myocardial infarction.
- Wolff–Parkinson–White syndrome.

Dosage
Oral
Loading
  200 mg t.i.d. (1 week). 200 mg b.d. (1 week).
Maintenance
  200 mg or less daily.
Intravenous bolus
  150–300 mg in 10–20 ml 5% dextrose over 1–2 minutes.
Infusion
  5 mg/kg over 20 minutes to 2 hours (dilute in 250 ml 5% dextrose) followed by up to 15 mg/kg every 24 hours if indicated.
NB
— Its use is contraindicated in sinus bradycardia, AV block and hypotensive states.
— Care should be taken when using it in combination with beta-blocking drugs or calcium antagonists as their action may be potentiated.
— The action of warfarin is potentiated.
— The plasma concentration of digoxin is increased.
— Thyroid disease is a relative contraindication.
— Thyroid function should be checked before and regularly during treatment. Reverse T_3 is increased.
— Pulmonary fibrosis and hepatotoxicity have been reported.

3.   Atropine

Uses and dosage
- Sinus bradycardia of haemodynamic significance.
  Intravenous bolus
      0.3–0.6 mg i.v. repeated as necessary.
- Prior to neostigmine in reversal of competitive neuromuscular blockade.
  Intravenous bolus
      0.6–1.2 mg.

NB
Narrow-angle glaucoma can be precipitated in susceptible individuals.

4. Bretylium tosylate

Use and dosage
Resistant ventricular dysrhythmias.
Intramuscular/intravenous bolus
  5–10 mg/kg repeated after 1–2 hours if necessary. Further doses of 5–10 mg/kg may be given at 6–8-hourly intervals for up to 5 days.

NB
— Bretylium may not exert its effect for some 20 minutes.
— The dose should be reduced in renal impairment.
— Its use is contraindicated in digitalis toxicity.
— An increase in blood pressure, heart rate and a positive inotropic effect may occur at the start of therapy. Hypotension is not uncommon once therapy is established.

5. Digoxin

Uses
• Atrial fibrillation and other supraventricular tachycardias.
• 'Heart failure'.

Dosage for digitalization
Rapid oral
  0.75–1.5 mg as a single dose.
  0.25 mg 6-hourly thereafter until a satisfactory heart rate is achieved.
Slow oral
  0.25–0.75 mg/day.
Intravenous
  0.5–1.0 mg (slowly) followed by 0.5 mg 4–6-hourly.
  Alternatively, an intravenous bolus of 0.125 mg can be administered hourly.
Maintenance
  0.125–0.25 mg/day.

Therapeutic range
1.3–2.5 nmol/litre.
Toxicity is suggested by nausea and vomiting, atrial and ventricular dysrhythmias and, occasionally, by bradycardia and atrioventricular block.
NB
— Hypokalaemia, hypomagnesaemia, hypercalcaemia and impaired renal function predispose to digoxin toxicity.
— The level of maintenance dosage should be reduced in the elderly.
— Concomitant use of quinidine and verapamil can also produce digoxin toxicity.

6. Disopyramide

Uses and dosage
Control of supraventricular and ventricular dysrhythmias.
Intravenous bolus
    2 mg/kg to a maximum of 150 mg over 5 minutes. Repeat once after 15 minutes if no response.
Infusion
    20–30 mg/hour to a maximum of 800 mg/day (10 mg/ml in a 5 ml ampoule).
Oral maintenance
    200 mg orally immediately on cessation of intravenous administration followed by 200 mg every 8 hours for 24 hours and 400–600 mg/day thereafter.
NB
— Care should be taken in patients with heart failure because of its marked negative inotropic effect.
— Its administration together with other negative inotropic drugs is not recommended.
— The dose should be reduced in patients with significant hepatic or renal impairment.

7. Edrophonium

Use and dosage
Control of supraventricular tachycardia.
Intravenous bolus
    5–10 mg slowly.
NB
Care should be taken when giving it to digitalized patients because of an increased risk of profound bradycardia.

8. Flecainide

Uses
- Prophylaxis of ventricular dysrhythmias.
- Treatment of certain forms of pre-excitation/nodal tachycardias.

Dosage
Intravenous bolus
  2 mg/kg over not less than 10 minutes.
  Maximum 150 mg.
Infusion (dilute in 5% dextrose)
  Start with a bolus of 2 mg/kg over 30 minutes and then give 1.5 mg/kg hour^{-1} for the first hour followed by 0.25 mg/kg hour^{-1} for subsequent hours.
Oral maintenance
  100 mg p.o. followed by 100–200 mg b.d. The infusion may be gradually discontinued over 4 hours following the initial oral dose.

NB
— Care should be taken in patients with heart failure because of its negative inotropic effect.
— It increases plasma digoxin levels by approximately 15%.

9. Glucagon

Use and dosage
As a positive inotropic agent in heart failure particularly in patients who are receiving β-blocking drugs.
Infusion
  4 mg (4 ampoules)/hour in 5% dextrose.
NB
Nausea and hyperglycaemia can occur.

10. Hydralazine

Use and dosage
Hypertensive crises.
Intravenous bolus
  20–40 mg slowly, repeated if necessary.

11.   Isosorbide dinitrate

Uses
- Preload and afterload reduction in acute left ventricular failure.
- Treatment of unstable angina pectoris.

Dosage
Sublingual
   5–10 mg p.r.n.
Infusion
   2–10 mg/hour.
NB
— Blood pressure should be frequently or continuously monitored.
— Isosorbide should not be administered via sets made of polyvinyl chloride.

Isosorbide dinitrate infusion regimens

	mg/hour	15 drops/ml	20 drops/ml	60 drops/ml
5 ampoules	1	2–3	3	10
isosorbide	2	5	7	20
dinitrate/	3	7–8	10	30
500 ml =	4	10	13	40
100 µg/ml	5	12.5	17	50
	6	15	20	60
	7	17–18	23	70
	8	20	27	80
	9	22–23	30	90
	10	25	33	100
10 ampoules	1	2	2	5
isosorbide	2	2–3	3	10
dinitrate/	3	4	5	15
500 ml =	4	5	7	20
200 µg/ml	5	6	8	25
	6	7–8	10	30
	7	9	12	35
	8	10	13	40
	9	11	15	45
	10	12–13	17	50

12. Labetalol

Uses
- Treatment of hypertension and hypertensive crises.
- Controlled hypotension.

Dosage
Oral
   100–200 mg b.d. increasing to 2.4 g/day.
Intravenous bolus
   50 mg over 1 minute repeated after 5 minutes if necessary
   up to a maximum of 200 mg.
   An ideal mixture is to add 200 mg of labetalol (40 ml) to
   10 ml of 5% dextrose and administer this by infusion pump.
Infusion
   2 mg/min up to a maximum of 200 mg/min.
Hypertension of pregnancy
   20 mg/hour doubled every 30 minutes to a maximum of
   160 mg/hour.

NB
— It should not be administered to patients with heart block.
— A history of asthma is a relative contraindication.
— The dose should be reduced in patients with significant
   hepatic impairment.

13. Lignocaine

Use and dosage
Ventricular dysrhythmias.
Intravenous bolus
   100 mg (5 ml Xylocard — 20 mg/ml).
Infusion
   4 mg/min for 12 hours and 2 mg/min for 12 hours and then
   discontinue.
If a smaller volume is required, 40 ml 2% = 800 mg should be
used as a neat solution and administered via a 50 ml infusion
pump at the appropriate setting.
NB
Lignocaine can precipitate convulsions in high dosage.

Lignocaine infusion regimens

	drops/min	15 drops/ml	20 drops/ml	60 drops/ml
		mg/min	mg/min	mg/min
200 mg/	1	0.026	0.02	0.0065
500 ml =	2	0.05	0.04	0.0125
0.4 mg/ml	5	0.13	0.1	0.025
	10	0.26	0.2	0.065
	15	0.4	0.3	0.1
	20	0.53	0.4	0.133
	40	1.07	0.8	0.27
	60	1.6	1.2	0.4
	75	2.0	1.5	0.5
	100	2.7	2.0	0.675
1000 mg/	1	0.13	0.1	0.0325
500 ml =	2	0.25	0.2	0.0525
2 mg/ml	5	0.65	0.5	0.125
	10	1.3	1.0	0.325
	15	2.0	1.5	0.5
	20	2.65	2.0	0.665
	40	5.35	4.0	1.35
	60	8.0	6.0	2.0
	75	10.0	7.5	2.5
	100	13.5	10.0	3.375

14.   Mexiletine hydrochloride

Use and dosage
Ventricular dysrhythmias especially following acute
myocardial infarction.
Loading dose
    100–250 mg i.v. over 5–10 minutes.
Infusion
    250 mg over 1 hour or 250 mg over 2 hours (500 mg in 500 ml
    5% dextrose/normal saline).
Intravenous maintenance
    0.5 mg/min according to response.
Oral maintenance
    200–250 mg t.i.d. on discontinuing infusion.
NB
Central nervous system and gastrointestinal side-effects
predominate.

15. Nitroglycerine

Uses
- Unstable angina.
- Preload and afterload reduction in acute left ventricular failure.
- Myocardial ischaemia during and post cardiovascular surgery.

Dosage
Sublingual
    0.3–1.0 mg p.r.n.
Topical
    5–20 mg p.r.n.
Infusion
    10–200 μg/min.
If a 50 ml infusion pump is to be used, 20 mg of nitroglycerine (40 ml) should be diluted with 10 ml of 5% dextrose to make up a concentration of 400 μg/ml and the pump should be adjusted to the required setting.

16. Phentolamine

Uses
- Preload and afterload reduction in acute left ventricular failure.
- Treatment of paroxysmal hypertension.

Dosage
Infusion
    5.0–60 mg over 10–30 minutes at a rate of 0.1–2.0 mg/min.

17. Phenytoin

Use and dosage
Ventricular dysrhythmias especially if digitalis toxicity is possible and in torsades de pointes:
Intravenous bolus
    5 mg/kg at 50 mg/min. Repeat once if necessary.
NB
Isoniazid, cimetidine, chloramphenicol and sulphonamides inhibit its metabolism.
Carbamazepine increases its clearance.

18.   **Practolol**

Use
Supraventricular dysrhythmias.

Dosage
Intravenous bolus
   5–10 mg repeated to a maximum of 20 mg.
NB
Particular care should be taken in patients with a history of
asthma, chronic obstructive airways disease or on verapamil
therapy.

19.   **Propafenone** (requires further clinical evaluation)

Use
Complex atrial and ventricular dysrhythmias

Dosage
Intravenous bolus
   450 mg.
Oral maintenance
   900 mg daily.
NB
—   No therapeutic range delineated.
—   Induced conduction defects and proarrhythmic effects
     described.

20.   **Sodium nitroprusside**

Uses
•   Afterload reduction in acute left ventricular failure.
•   Hypertensive crises.
•   To induce hypotension in surgical procedures.

Dosage
Infusion
   0.5 μg/kg min^{-1} to a maximum of 800 μg/min.
   (ECG and blood pressure monitoring is essential.)

Infusion regimens
As soon as the infusion solution is prepared the burette

should be wrapped in aluminium foil to prevent the sodium nitroprusside being degraded by light.

	drops/min	15 drops/ml	20 drops/ml	60 drops/ml
		µg/min	µg/min	µg/min
50 mg	1	6.7	5	1.67
(2 ml)/	2	13.0	10	3.4
500 ml 5%	3	20.0	15	5.0
dextrose =	4	26.7	20	6.7
100 µg/ml	5	33.0	25	8.3
	6	40.0	30	10.0
	7	46.7	35	11.7
	8	53.3	40	13.3
	9	60.0	45	15.0
	10	67.0	50	16.7
50 mg	1	3.35	2.5	0.835
(2ml)/	2	6.5	5.0	1.7
1 litre 5%	3	10.0	7.5	2.5
dextrose =	4	13.25	10.0	3.35
50 µg/ml	5	17.5	12.5	4.15
	6	20.0	15.0	5.0
	7	23.35	17.5	5.85
	8	26.55	20.0	6.65
	9	30.0	22.5	7.5
	10	33.5	25.0	8.35

If a smaller volume is required, dilute 50 mg (2 ml) in 48 ml of 5% dextrose and administer via a 50 ml infusion pump (1 mg/ml) at the appropriate setting.
NB
— Sodium nitroprusside is converted to cyanide and thiocyanate; therefore if high infusion rates are used, there is a danger of metabolic acidosis and cyanide toxicity.
— Particular care should be taken in the elderly.

21. Sympathomimetic drugs

1. Adrenaline.
2. Dobutamine.
3. Dopamine.
4. Isoprenaline.
5. Noradrenaline.

Uses

Correction of poor perfusion, low cardiac output,
impending renal failure and 'shock' associated with:
— Myocardial infarction.
— Trauma (after hypovolaemia has been corrected).
— Septicaemia.
— Open heart surgery.
— Acute heart failure of other causes.

Receptors

α_1 — Constriction of peripheral and visceral vessels.
        Bladder and uterine contraction.
α_2 — Inhibition of catecholamine release from nerve endings.
        Dilatation in vessels with sympathetically mediated
        tone.
β_1 — Increase in myocardial contractility and heart rate.
        Lipolysis.
        Increase in renin output.
β_2 — Bronchodilatation.
        Skeletal muscle and coronary arteriolar
        vasodilatation.
        Uterine relaxation.
        Gluconeogenesis.
Dopaminergic — Increase in myocardial contractility.
             — Dilatation of renal, coronary and
                mesenteric arterioles.

Actions	Adrenaline	Dobutamine	Dopamine	Isoprenaline	Noradrenaline
Cardiac output	↑	↑	↑ Dose dependent	↑	Insignificant
Heart rate	↑	↑ Minimal	↑ Dose dependent	↑	↓
Contractility	↑	↑	↑	↑	↑ Minimal
Tachydysrhythmia	↑	↑ Low incidence	↑	↑	↑
Total peripheral resistance	↑ Dose dependent	↑	↑ Dose dependent	↓	↑
Mean arterial pressure	↑	↑	↑ ↑	↓	↑
Fractional renal blood flow			↑		

(i)   Adrenaline

Dosage

Infusion

Commence at 0.3 μg/kg min^{-1} (approximately 2.0 μg/min for a 70 kg man = 15 standard drops/min).

Infusion regimens

	drops/min	15 drops/ml	20 drops/ml	60 drops/ml
		μg/min	μg/min	μg/min
1 ml of	1	0.13	0.1	0.333
1:1000 or	2	0.26	0.2	0.065
10 ml of	5	0.65	0.5	0.162
1:10 000/	10	1.3	1.0	0.32
500 ml =	15	2.0	1.5	0.5
2 μg/ml	20	2.6	2.0	0.65
	40	5.2	4.0	1.33
	60	7.8	6.5	2.0
	75	9.75	7.5	2.44
	100	13.0	10.0	3.25
2 ml of	1	0.26	0.2	0.66
1:1000 or	2	0.52	0.4	0.130
20 ml of	5	1.3	1.0	0.324
1:10000/	10	2.6	2.0	0.64
500 ml =	15	4.0	3.0	1.0
4 μg/ml	20	5.2	4.0	1.30
	40	10.4	8.0	2.6
	60	15.6	13.0	4.0
	75	19.5	15.0	4.88
	100	26.0	20.0	6.50

If a 50 ml infusion pump is to be used, 2 ml of 1:1000 adrenaline (2 mg) should be added to 48 ml of 5% dextrose to make up a concentration of 40 μg/ml and the infusion pump should be adjusted to the appropriate setting.

(ii)   Dobutamine

Dosage

Infusion

Commence at 2.5 μg/kg min^{-1} — 10 μg/kg min^{-1} to a maximum of 40 μg/kg min^{-1}.

Infusion regimen

Add 2 × 250 mg dobutamine in 500 ml i.v. solution = 1000 μg/ml and administer by infusion according to the tables below.

Standard giving set 15 drops/ml			
Body weight (kg)	Dose (μg/kg min^{-1})		
	2.5	5.0	7.5	10.0

Body weight (kg)	2.5	5.0	7.5	10.0
40	2	3	5	6
50	2	4	6	8
60	2	5	7	9
70	3	5	8	11
80	3	6	9	12
90	3	7	10	14
100	4	8	11	15
110	4	8	12	17
120	5	9	14	18

Standard giving set 20 drops/ml

Dose (μg/kg min^{-1})

Body weight (kg)	2.5	5.0	7.5	10.0
40	2	4	6	8
50	2	5	7	10
60	3	6	9	12
70	3	7	10	14
80	4	8	12	16
90	4	9	13	18
100	5	10	15	20
110	5	11	16	22
120	6	12	18	24

Paediatric giving set 60 ml/min

Dose (μg/kg min^{-1})

Body weight (kg)	2.5	5.0	7.5	10.0
40	6	12	18	24
50	7	15	22	30
60	9	18	27	36
70	10	21	31	42
80	12	24	36	48
90	13	27	40	54
100	15	30	45	60
110	16	33	49	66
120	18	36	54	72

(iii)   Dopamine

Dosage range

1–5 μg/kg min^{-1}
  increased glomerular filtration rate (GFR), renal blood
  flow, sodium excretion and urine output.

5–20 μg/kg min^{-1}
  increased cardiac output and arterial pressure.

20+ μg/kg min^{-1}
  increased arterial pressure and constriction of the renal
  and mesenteric vessels.

Infusion regimen

Add 800 mg (4 × 5 ml ampoules) to 500 ml intravenous
solution and administer by infusion according to the
following tables. If a lower volume is required, add 200 mg
dopamine to 45 ml 5% dextrose and administer by a 50 ml
infusion pump at the appropriate setting.

	Standard giving set at 15 drops/ml			
Body weight	Dose (μg/kg min^{-1})			
(kg)	2.0	5.0	10.0	20.0
40	1	2	4	8
50	1	2	5	10
60	1	3	6	12
70	1	3	7	14
80	1	4	8	16
90	2	4	9	17
100	2	5	10	19
110	2	5	11	21
120	2	6	12	23

	Standard giving set at 20 drops/ml			
Body weight	Dose (μg/kg min^{-1})			
(kg)	2.0	5.0	10.0	20.0
40	1	3	5	10
50	1	3	7	13
60	2	4	8	18
70	2	5	9	18
80	2	5	10	21
90	2	6	12	23
100	3	7	13	26
110	3	7	14	29
120	3	8	16	31

Paediatric giving set at 60 drops/ml				
Body weight (kg)	Dose (μg/kg min^{-1})			
	2.0	5.0	10.0	20.0
40	3	8	16	31
50	4	10	20	39
60	5	12	23	47
70	5	14	27	55
80	6	16	31	62
90	7	18	35	70
100	8	20	39	78
110	9	21	43	86
120	9	23	47	94

(iv) Isoprenaline

Dosage
Infusion commence at 1 μg/min.

Infusion regimens

	drops/min	15 drops/ml	20 drops/ml	60 drops/ml
		μg/min	μg/min	μg/min
2.0 mg/ 500 ml = 4 μg/ml	1	0.26	0.2	0.666
	2	0.52	0.4	0.132
	5	1.3	1.0	0.33
	10	2.6	2.0	0.66
	15	4.0	3.0	0.99
	20	5.2	4.0	1.32
	40	10.4	8.0	2.64
	60	15.6	12.0	4.0
	75	19.5	15.0	4.95
	100	26.0	20.0	6.6
5.0 mg/ 500 ml = 10 μg/ml	1	0.7	0.5	0.16
	2	1.3	1.0	0.4
	5	3.3	2.5	0.8
	10	6.7	5.0	1.6
	15	10.0	7.5	2.5
	20	13.0	10.0	3.3
	40	26.0	20.0	6.6
	60	40.0	30.0	10.0
	75	50.0	37.5	12.5
	100	66.7	50.0	16.6

If a 50 ml infusion pump is to be used, 2 ml of isoprenaline should be added to 48 ml of 5% dextrose to make up a concentration of 40 μg/ml and the pump should be adjusted to the appropriate setting.

(v)   Noradrenaline

Dosage
Infusion
    1.0–12.0 μg/min, i.e. 8 mg (2 × 2 ml ampoules) in 250 ml
    5% dextrose at 2–20 microdrops/min.

22.   Tocainide hydrochloride

Use and dosage
Treatment of life threatening dysrhythmias associated with poor left ventricular function resistant to other therapy.
Infusion
    500–750 mg over 20 min followed by 600–800 mg p.o.
Oral maintenance
    400 mg t.i.d.
NB
—   Blood dyscrasias usually in the first 12 weeks of
    treatment. Regular blood counts recommended.
—   The dose should be reduced in patients with significant
    hepatic or renal impairment.

23.   Trimetaphan camsylate

Use and dosage
Controlled hypotension:
Infusion
    Commence at 3 mg/min (e.g. 250 mg ampoule in 250 ml
    5% dextrose or normal saline at 60 drops/min via a 20
    drops/ml pump).

24.   Verapamil

Use and dosage
Supraventricular dysrhythmias including those associated with the Wolff–Parkinson–White syndrome:
Intravenous bolus
    5 mg slowly over 30 seconds to a maximum of 20 mg over
    15 minutes.

NB
i.v. verapamil should not be administered concurrently to patients taking either i.v. or oral β-blocking drugs.

Techniques

1. Elective cardioversion

Indications
— Atrial flutter.
— Atrial fibrillation:
  ○ Uncontrolled by medical therapy.
  ○ With a history of peripheral emboli.
  ○ In treated thyrotoxicosis.
— Supraventricular tachycardia unresponsive to medical therapy with a compromised haemodynamic state.

Equipment
— Standard resuscitative apparatus.
— Synchronized DC defibrillator.

Procedure
• Obtain consent.
• If necessary, transfer the patient to a high dependency monitoring area.
• Request the presence of an anaesthetist.
• Ensure digoxin has been withheld for at least 24–48 hours.
• Ensure anticoagulation has been instituted if necessary.
• Sedate patient as appropriate (e.g. intravenous diazepam, brietal, midazolam).
• Check that the synchronizer is on and place paddles over the 5th left intercostal space in the midclavicular line and the 2nd left intercostal space at the sternal edge.
  Commence with a low energy shock, e.g. 50 watt seconds (WS). Increase in steps of 50 WS as necessary.

Relative contraindication
Digoxin toxicity.

Complications
— Embolization following restoration of sinus rhythm.
— Cardiac dysrhythmias; asystole.

2. Temporary transvenous pacing

Indications
— 3° atrioventricular (AV) block.
— Mobitz type 2 2° AV block.
— Mobitz type 1 2° AV block complicating anterior myocardial infarction.
— Ventricular conduction defects in acute myocardial infarction.
    Strong indications*:
        Long PR interval and new right bundle branch block (RBBB) plus left posterior hemi-block (LPHB).
        Long PR interval and new RBBB plus left anterior hemi-block (LAHB).
        Alternating RBBB and left bundle branch block (LBBB).
    Moderately strong indications:
        Long PR interval and LBBB.
        Normal PR interval and RBBB plus LPHB.
    Weak indications:
        Normal PR interval and RBBB plus LAHB.
        Normal PR interval and LBBB.
— Sinoatrial disease post myocardial infarction if associated with significant sinus bradycardia, sinus arrest or sinus exit block that is not responsive to atropine.
— Overdosage (e.g. digoxin).
— Refractory tachyarrhythmias.

Equipment
— Pacing wire box.
— Electrocardiogram (ECG) monitor.
— Full resuscitation apparatus.
— Intravenous introducer — see insertion of a catheter sheath (page 29).
— Appropriate screening facilities.

Procedure
• Transfer the patient to a suitable screening room in the X-ray department or arrange for use of a portable image intensifier.
• Ensure that full resuscitation facilities are available.

- Set 5° downward tilt on table allowing patient one pillow and prepare and towel insertion site.
- Perform central venous catheterization (page 27).
- Thread pacing wire carefully through catheter sheath. Wire should run smoothly with no resistance.
- Once the wire has been advanced approximately 6–8 cm, withdraw catheter sheath over the pacing wire to a more proximal position and apply pressure for a minute or so at the entry point.
- Screen and advance wire to the right atrial margin then continue to advance because the wire often attains a satisfactory right ventricular position with no special manipulation (Fig. 1.1, position 1).

    The wire tip should tend to point downwards and not float high in the right ventricular outflow tract or pulmonary artery.

Potential problems

    ○ Wire persistently travels down inferior vena cava or hepatic veins (Fig. 1.1, position 2).

    Solution

    Impact wire at the right atrial margin (Fig. 1.1, position 3).

    Continue to advance so that a loop is formed (Fig. 1.1, position 4).

    Rotate wire through 180° and then slowly withdraw. The wire will flip into the right ventricle and can be advanced in the usual way.

    ○ Wire enters coronary sinus and not right ventricle (easy to do!)

    Solution

    Withdraw the wire into the superior vena cava and reinsert.

    Placement in the coronary sinus can be confirmed as the wire will not advance.

    ○ Wire will not enter right ventricular cavity despite extensive manipulation.

    Solution

    Remove the wire, manually bend the terminal few centimeters into a gentle curve and reintroduce.

- Once its position is stable, connect the proximal end to

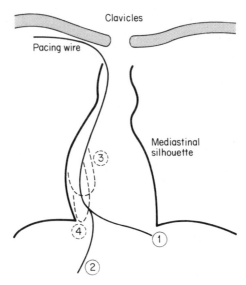

Fig. 1.1   Possible positions of pacing wire. 1. satisfactory right ventricular position; 2, wire in inferior vena cava or a hepatic vein; 3, wire impacted in right atrial margin; 4, wire advanced from position 3 to form a loop.

the pacing box ensuring that distal is + (active) and proximal is − (indifferent). Set controls as:
   1.   Demand.
   2.   Rate, approximately 70/min.
   3.   Voltage, approximately 2 volts.

Then check that ventricular pacing is occurring. If the ventricles do not 'capture' at 2 volts then the wire needs repositioning.

• Once repositioned reduce the pacing voltage until the ventricles no longer capture. The voltage at which this occurs is the 'threshold'. Set the voltage to the threshold + 2 volts and test its security by asking the patient to cough, pant and take deep breaths in succession whilst watching the monitor.

• Adequately secure the wire in position. A combination of silk sutures and external covering with 'Op-site' is suitable.

• Perform a chest X-ray (CXR) to exclude a pneumothorax.

- Check pacing threshold at least once daily and record the level in the notes.

Complications
— Pneumothorax in relation to subclavian vein puncture.
— Myocardial perforation:
    If the right ventricular wall is perforated the pacing threshold will rise, pacing may fail and a pericardial friction rub may appear. In this event, reposition the wire. If the interventricular septum is perforated, the ECG will change from an LBBB to an RBBB pattern; again reposition the wire.
— Infection:
    Remove the wire and insert a new one from the opposite side.
— Unacceptable rise in threshold:
    Exclude myocardial perforation (above), and reposition the wire.

Discontinuation of pacing
Heart block usually lasts less than a week following an acute myocardial infarction, but it can last up to 3 weeks. If heart block is still present at this time, a permanent pacemaker will need to be considered. When pacing has not been required for 24 hours, then the wire can be removed.

* Hayward, R. (1981). Who do we pace? *British Journal of Hospital Medicine* **25**, 466–74.

3. Central venous catheterization

Indications
— Central venous pressure measurement.
— Intravenous hyperalimentation (for insertion *see* p. 29).
— Drug and fluid administration in cardiac resuscitation.
— Cardiac pacing.

A. Infraclavicular percutaneous subclavian line

Equipment
— Sterile towels, gown, suture pack, gloves.
— Iodine solution or equivalent.
— 10 ml syringe, 2% lignocaine, No. 15 blade.

— 25G, 21G gauge needles.
— 2 × 30 silk sutures.
— 10 ml normal saline.
— Op-site or equivalent.
— Catheter (e.g. Leader-cath Vygon Codes 115-120-124).

Procedure
- Place the patient on a tilting bed/operating table 25° head down.
- Prepare the skin and towel (right side preferred). Turn the patient's head to the opposite side.
- Identify the right clavicle and sternomastoid.
- Identify the point of intended insertion of the cannula (immediately below clavicle at the junction of the middle and lateral thirds of the clavicle) and infiltrate with 2% lignocaine ensuring that the periosteum of the clavicle is anaesthetized.
- Fill introducing syringe with 2–5 ml of normal saline.
- Carefully introduce needle through skin and advance in a cephalad direction until the clavicle is touched. Place the index finger of your left hand in the patient's suprasternal notch. Swing the needle through approximately 70°, so that the needle points medially, and aim in the direction of the tip of your left index finger.
- Slowly advance the needle in the above direction ensuring that its upper surface 'scrapes' underneath the clavicle. Maintain a slight negative pressure on the syringe until the vein is entered as judged by easy aspiration of venous blood (Fig. 1.2, part 1).
- Hold the needle in position in the vessel and rotate it through 90° so that the bevel is now pointing downwards.
- Remove the syringe and pass the guide wire through the needle advancing the flexible tip (guilded) first (Fig. 1.2, part 2).
- Withdraw the needle over the guide wire leaving the wire *in situ* (Fig. 1.2, parts 3 and 4).
- Make a small incision (No. 15 blade) in the skin where the guide wire leaves the skin (Fig. 1.2, part 5). Thread the catheter over the wire so that the wire protrudes over the end and gradually advance the catheter until in position (Fig. 1.2, part 6).

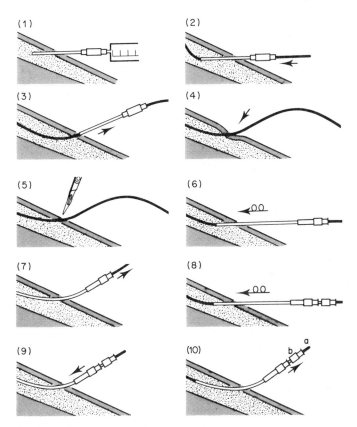

Fig. 1.2 Stages in inserting a central venous catheter by the Seldinger technique.

1, vascular puncture; 2, introduction of the guide wire; 3 and 4, removal of the needle; 5, incision where the guide wire leaves the skin; 6 and 7, introduction of the catheter (for full details of this procedure *see* text, page 28).

Insertion of a catheter sheath.

8, introduction of the dilator into the vessel; 9, entry of sheath into vessel; 10, removal of guide wire and dilator (for full details of this procedure *see* text, page 30).

- Remove the guide wire (Fig. 1.2, part 7). Fix the catheter to the skin and attach the appropriate CVP monitoring apparatus.

Relative contraindications
— Pneumonectomy on opposite side.
— Pneumothorax on opposite side.
— Bleeding diathesis.

B.   Insertion of a catheter sheath for pacing wire, flotation catheter or feeding line

Additional equipment
— Substitute catheter for a catheter sheath (e.g. Desilet introducer — Vygon).

Procedure
- The first ten procedures as for infraclavicular line.
- Thread the dilator and catheter over the guide wire together and advance with a gentle rotation (Fig. 1.2, parts 8 and 9).
- Once in place, remove the guide wire (Fig. 1.2, part 10a) and then the dilator (Fig. 1.2, part 10b).
- A pacing wire or feeding line can then be threaded through the catheter sheath.

C.   Insertion of a subclavian line by a tunnelling technique

Additional equipment
— Silicone intravenous catheter for long-term parenteral nutrition (e.g. Nutricath 'S' Vygon).

Procedure
- Complete the procedure for insertion of a catheter sheath (*see* above).
- Cut the silicone catheter to the required length (estimate this by surface markings) and thread down the catheter sheath with a rotating motion.
- Whilst advancing the catheter start to withdraw the stilette.
- Once the catheter is in position remove the stilette and catheter sheath leaving the catheter *in situ*; attach hub, and flush with 5 ml of normal saline.

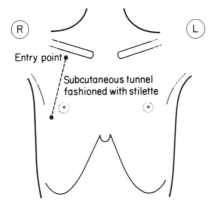

Fig. 1.3 Site of subcutaneous tunnel for subclavian line.

- Create a subcutaneous tunnel, approximately 10 cm long, away from the entry point (the introducing stilette in the above Nutricath 'S' is a useful implement for this manoeuvre) (Fig. 1.3).
- Remove the hub from the end of the catheter and feed the catheter through the stilette sheath (Fig. 1.4).
- Pull the catheter taut so that it is no longer visible at the entry site and reattach the hub.
- Suture the hub to the skin, attach appropriate extension tube and cover with Op-site.
- Confirm the position of the catheter tip by chest X-ray.

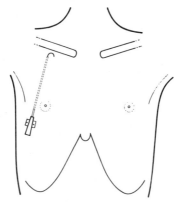

Fig. 1.4 Subclavian line in position.

D. Internal jugular vein cannulation (lateral approach)

Additional equipment
— Intravenous cannula (e.g. 13.3 cm 16GA Angiocath).

Procedure
- Place the patient on a tilting bed/operating table 25° head down.
- Prepare the skin, towel and turn the patient's head to the left; cannulation of the right side is preferred:
  ○ To avoid damaging the thoracic duct.
  ○ Because the route of cannulation is direct to the right atrium).
- Insert the needle, with a saline-filled syringe attached, along the lateral border of the sternomastoid, just proximal to where the external jugular vein crosses it (Fig. 1.5).
  The carotid artery lies medial to this.
  Elevate the needle approximately 10° above the coronal plane and aim for the sternal notch advancing the needle underneath the sternomastoid. The internal jugular vein is entered after approximately 6 cm.
- Once the vein is entered inject saline as the cannula is advanced over the needle (Angiocath) or, alternatively,

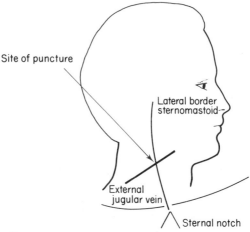

Site of puncture

Lateral border
sternomastoid

External
jugular vein

Sternal notch

Fig. 1.5 Entry site for internal jugular cannulation.

insert a Seldinger wire over which a catheter can be inserted.

Complications of all routes of insertion
— Pneumothorax.
— Accidental arterial puncture.
— Septicaemia.
— Thrombosis (case for intravenous heparin 5000 iu 12-hourly).
— Air embolism.
— Myocardial perforation (very rare with subclavian punctures).
— Catheter embolus (very rare with modern techniques).

4. Arterial line insertion

Indications
— Continuous arterial pressure monitoring.
— When frequent arterial blood samples are needed (e.g. for blood gas analysis).

A. Radial artery cannulation

Equipment
— Sterile towels, gown, suture pack, gloves.
— Iodine solution or equivalent.
— 5 ml syringe, 1% lignocaine, No. 15 blade.
— 25G, 21G needles.
— Arterial cannula (e.g. 20G Abbocath).
— Tape.
— Arterial line plus transducing apparatus already primed with solution (e.g. normal saline).

Procedure
• Check platelet count and coagulation status.
• Check the adequacy of the collateral circulation between ulnar and radial artery by compressing both arteries for 2–3 minutes and then releasing the ulnar compression only. If an adequate collateral circulation is present, the whole hand should flush within a few seconds* (Fig. 1.6).
• Select arterial cannula.

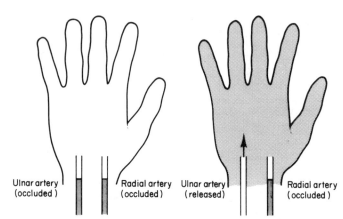

Fig. 1.6   Confirmation of adequacy of collateral circulation.

- Prepare the skin and infiltrate with 1% lignocaine on each side of the artery in question.
- Break the skin with the No. 15 blade over intended site of puncture.
- Extend the wrist slightly.
- Advance the cannula, with the bevel uppermost, along the line of the artery which is palpable with the middle and index finger of the nondominant hand at 30° to the skin surface until the artery is entered, as demonstrated by 'flashback' into the cannula.
- Lower the angle of insertion to 10–20°, and carefully advance cannula and needle a further 4 mm. Then advance the cannula off the needle.
- Remove the needle and attach the already primed arterial line.
- Tape the line into place.

B.   Femoral artery cannulation

Equipment
— Sterile towels, gown, suture pack and gloves.
— Iodine solution or equivalent.
— 5 ml syringe, 1% lignocaine, No. 15 blade.
— 25G, 21G needles.
— Arterial cannula (e.g. Leader–Cath–Vygon).
— 2 × 30 silk sutures.

— 10 ml normal saline.
— Tape.
— Arterial line plus transducing apparatus already primed with solution (e.g. normal saline).

Procedure
• Check platelet count and coagulation status.
• Select arterial cannula.
• Prepare and towel area around left/right common femoral artery having first assessed the adequacy of the femoral, dorsalis pedis and popliteal pulses bilaterally.
• Infiltrate deep to both sides of the common femoral artery with 1% lignocaine.
• Fill introducing syringe with 2–5 ml normal saline.
• Percutaneously puncture the common femoral artery at an angle of 45° to the skin surface and insert the guide wire with the gilt edge foremost (Fig. 1.2, parts 1–7), once satisfactory backflow is achieved.
• Withdraw the needle over the guide wire, leaving the wire *in situ*.
• Make a small incision (No. 15 blade) in the skin where the guide wire leaves the skin. Thread the catheter over the wire so that the wire protrudes over the end and gradually advance the catheter until it is in position.
• Remove the guide wire and suture the catheter to the skin.

Complications
— Haemorrhage/thrombosis.
— Infection.
— Vascular insufficiency.
— Fistula formation.
— Aneurysm formation.
— Dissection.

* Allen, EV. (1929) Thromboangiitis obliterans; methods of diagnosis of chronic occlusive arterial lesions distal to wrist with illustrative cases. *American Journal of Medical Science*, **178**, 237–44.

5.   Insertion of a flow-directed flotation catheter

Indications
— Measurement of pulmonary capillary wedge pressure (PCWP).
— Measurement of cardiac output.
— Investigation and management of pulmonary hypertension, particularly in patients with suspected pulmonary embolism.
— Diagnosis of pericardial tamponade.
— Diagnosis of acute ventricular septal defect (VSD), mitral incompetence.

Equipment
— 'Swan–Ganz' flow-directed catheter size 6FG, 7FG or equivalent.
— Model 9520A cardiac output computer or equivalent.
— Monitoring and resuscitation equipment (e.g. ECG, pressure transducer, 'intraflo' or equivalent flush system, defibrillator and 'cardiac arrest' equipment).
— Central venous catheterization equipment (page 27).

Procedure
• Decide whether the simple two lumina catheter or the quadruple lumen design thermodilution catheter is indicated.
• Prime the monitoring lumina with normal saline.
• Ensure:
  ○ That the balloon fills satisfactorily by introducing the required volume of air into the lumen.
  ○ That the catheter and balloon fit through the chosen cannula.
• Slowly advance the catheter into the thoracic veins following insertion of a catheter sheath (page 30) and attach a pressure transducer. Entry of the catheter and tip into the thorax is associated with an increased respiratory fluctuation in pressure.
  Note the distance the catheter has been advanced:
  Right atrium (RA)/   = 40 cm from right
  Superior vena cava   antecubital fossa.
  (SVC) junction

RA/Inferior vena cava (IVC) junction	= 50 cm from left antecubital fossa.
	= 15-20 cm from right subclavian/internal jugular vein.
	= 30 cm from femoral vein.

Then inflate the balloon.

Observe the pressure waveforms and advance the catheter with the balloon inflated through the right atrium, right ventricle, into the pulmonary artery and into the wedge position (Fig. 1.7).

- Once PCWP is achieved deflate the balloon to ensure the tracing returns to pulmonary artery pressure (PAP).
- Secure the catheter in position with sutures. 'Op-site' is useful.
- Check catheter position with a penetrated CXR.

Problems

- Difficulty in obtaining PCWP.
  Solution:
    Deflate the balloon, withdraw catheter into the right atrium and repeat the procedure.
- Failure to enter right ventricle (RV) or pulmonary artery (PA).
  Solution:
  ○ If appropriate, ask the patient to take a deep inspiration during catheter advancement.
  ○ Slowly perfuse the catheter with 5-10 ml of sterile normal saline as the catheter is advanced.
  ○ Use a 7FG rather than a 6FG catheter.

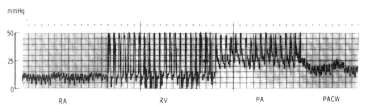

Fig. 1.7 Pressure waveforms during insertion of a flotation catheter.
RA, right atrium; RV, right ventricle; PA, pulmonary artery; PACW, pulmonary artery capillary wedge.

- Ventricular dysrhythmia — this is usually caused by the catheter recoiling towards the pulmonary valve or slipping into the right ventricle when the balloon is deflated.
  Solution:
     Reinflate the balloon and advance the catheter by 2–3 cm.
- Spontaneous wedging — as the catheter material softens, the tip migrates into the smaller branches of the PA and wedges.
  Solution:
  ○ Ensure that the earliest wedging position is achieved.
  ○ Always withdraw the catheter 2–3 cm from the wedge position between readings.

Complications (uncommon)
— Pulmonary infarction.
— Thromboembolism.
— Sepsis/right-sided endocarditis.
— Kinking.
— Knotting.
— Stretching.
— Conduction/rhythm disturbances.
— Complications of insertion (*see* page 33).

— spurious wedging.

Interpretation
— Mean PCWP is approximately 1–4 mmHg less than pulmonary artery diastolic pressure (PADP).
— In acute mitral incompetence a large (v) wave is present in the recorded wedge pressure.
— In restrictive/constrictive heart disease the difference between PCWP in diastole and systole is reduced.
— In patients on a ventilator, with or without positive end expiratory pressure (PEEP) or with severe lung disease:
  true intracardiac pressure = measured intracardiac pressure − intrathoracic pressure.
— Conditions in which:
  PCWP > left ventricular end diastolic pressure (LVEDP)
  Mitral stenosis.
  Left atrial myxoma.

Pulmonary venous obstruction.
High intra-alveolar pressure.
PCWP < LVEDP
Stiff left ventricle.
High (> 25 mmHg) LVEDP.

A.   Determination of cardiac output (CO) by thermodilution

Principle
A known amount of saline at a set temperature (usually 0°C or room temperature) is injected into the right atrium via the catheter. The consequent change in blood temperature as a result of mixing is detected by a thermistor situated in the pulmonary artery. By computation using the Stewart–Hamilton equation CO is derived:

$$CO = \frac{CC\,(T_B - T_I)}{1.22\int_0^{t_\triangle} T_B(t)\,dt}$$

CO = Cardiac output (litres/min).
CC = Computation constant.
T_B = Initial blood temperature in °C.
T_I = Initial injectate temperature in °C.
$\int_0^{t_\triangle} T_B(t)\,dt$ = Area under the time–temperature
        thermodilution curve in °C from $0 \rightarrow t$.
t = Time at which amplitude of the thermodilution curve returns to 30% of peak amplitude.
1.22 = Correction factor for area under the thermodilution curve beyond t.

Procedure
- Consult appropriate manual for description of setting of CO computer and chart recorder.
- Connect catheter to computer.
- Prepare 10 10 ml syringes (5 ml if the volume is a problem) of 5% dextrose and suspend in an ice bath.
- Insert catheter into pulmonary artery.
- Check the patient's blood temperature is stable.
- Enter the appropriate computation constant into the computer.

- Rapidly inject (< 4 sec) contents of the syringe into the proximal catheter lumen with minimal handling. The resultant blood/injectate mixture temperature is recorded by the thermistor and the CO and thermodilution curves are automatically produced.
- Perform at least three serial measurements and obtain a mean value.

6.   Pericardial aspiration

Indications
— Elective.
  ○ For microscopy, culture (including alcohol and acid-fast bacilli), cytology, cells, protein content, sugar and rheumatoid factor in the pericardial fluid.
  ○ Insertion of cytotoxic agents and antibiotics into the pericardial sac.
— Emergency relief of cardiac tamponade.

Equipment
— Sterile towels, gown, suture pack and gloves.
— Iodine solution or equivalent.
— 5 ml syringe, 20 ml syringe, 1% lignocaine, No. 15 blade.
— 25G, 21G needles.
— 16FG intravenous cannula (e.g. Angiocath) or Seldinger wire and cannula or 18G LP needle.
— 2 × 30 silk sutures.
— 20 ml normal saline.
— Tape.
— ECG monitoring apparatus.
— Resuscitation facilities.
— Screening facilities, if available.

Procedure
- Group and save serum, if time permits.
- Gown, prepare and towel the patient whose chest should be positioned at 45° to the horizontal.
- Infiltrate the skin and subcutaneous tissue down to the pericardium at chosen entry site with 1% lignocaine (Fig. 1.8).

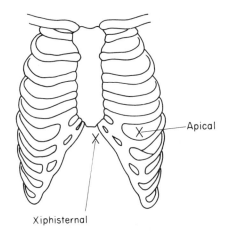

Fig. 1.8 Sites of insertion of needle for pericardial aspiration.

- If continuous ECG monitoring is to be used, attach precordial lead of ECG to LP needle with suitable sterile connection and set for V lead recording.
  The position of the tip of the needle can be determined by the ECG record:
  Skin   — Normal V1/V2 complexes.
  Ventricle — ST segment elevation + ventricular ectopics.
  Atrium   — Increase in size of P wave.
  An intravenous cannula or Seldinger wire and cannula is more suitable if a large amount or thick fluid is suspected.

Xiphisternal route
- Attach a three-way stopcock and a 20 ml syringe to the intravenous cannula.
- Make a small nick in the skin (e.g. use a No. 15 blade) at site of entry. Identify the angle between the xiphisternum and the left costal margin (Fig. 1.8).
- Position the cannula at 45° to the horizontal plane and advance slowly approximately 5° to the left of the midline, aiming for the tip of the left shoulder.
- Aspirate continuously.
- Once the pericardial sac is entered, advance the cannula

and withdraw the needle or insert the Seldinger wire under screening and then thread an appropriate cannula over it into the pericardial sac.

The wire can then be removed and the cannula secured.

Apical route
• Identify the apex beat and enter approximately 1.5 cm laterally and one costal space lower.
• Advance slowly aiming towards tip of right shoulder.
• Aspirate continuously.
• Once the effusion is entered, advance the cannula and withdraw the needle.

NB
Intracardiac blood clots — fluid aspirated from the pericardium does not.

Complications
— Dysrhythmias/death.
— Damage to:
  ◦ Left or right ventricle (Fig. 1.9).

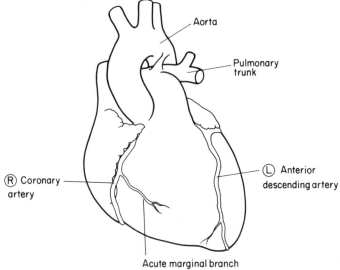

Fig. 1.9   Potential sites of cardiac damage following pericardial aspiration.

- ○ Right coronary artery or acute marginal branch (Xiphisternal approach).
- ○ Left anterior descending artery or branch (Apical approach).
- ○ Left lung.
- ○ Left internal mammary artery.
- ○ Liver.

2 Respiratory system

Data

1. Blood gas tensions and pH

— Arterial
pH: 7.36–7.44.
$[H^+]$: 36–44 nmol/litre.
Po_2: 85–100 mmHg (11.3–13.3 kPa).
Pco_2: 36–44 mmHg (4.8–5.9 kPa).
— Mixed venous
pH: 7.34–7.42.
$[H^+]$: 38–46 nmol/litre.
Po_2: 37–42 mmHg (5.0–5.6 kPa).
Pco_2: 42–50 mmHg (5.6–6.7 kPa).

2. Lung volumes (70 kg adult at rest) (Fig. 2.1)

Total lung capacity $\simeq$ 6.0 litres.
Tidal volume $\simeq$ 500 ml.
Inspiratory capacity $\simeq$ 3.6 litres.
Inspiratory reserve volume = 2.0–3.2 litres.
Expiratory reserve volume = 0.75–1.0 litres.
Vital capacity = 3.2–4.8 litres.
Residual volume = 1.2 litres.
Functional residual capacity = 1.95–2.2 litres.

3. Spirometry curves (Fig. 2.2)

After a deep inspiration the patient breathes out as
forcefully and as rapidly as possible. The volume of air
expired in the first second is denoted FEV_1 (forced

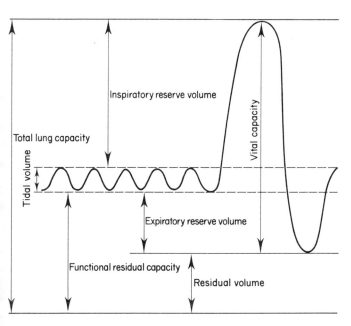

Fig. 2.1   Lung volumes for a 70 kg adult.

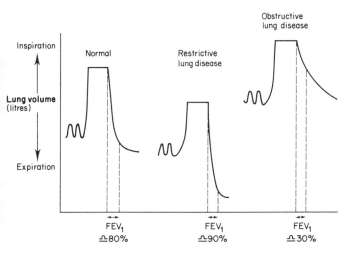

Fig. 2.2   Spirometry curves.

expiratory volume in one second). The total volume expired
is the vital capacity.

4. Oxygen consumption

$$\dot{V}O_2 = (\dot{V}I \times FIO_2) - (\dot{V}E \times FEO_2)$$
$$\simeq 250 \text{ ml/min}$$

$\dot{V}$ = Volume of gas/unit time.
F = Fractional concentration in dry gas.
I = Inspired.
E = Expired.
$\dot{V}O_2$ = Oxygen consumption.

5. Percentage venous admixture (shunt equation)

$$\frac{\dot{Q}S}{\dot{Q}T} = \frac{CcO_2 - CaO_2}{CcO_2 - C\bar{v}O_2} \simeq \frac{(PAO_2 - PaO_2) \times 0.0031}{(PAO_2 - PaO_2) \times 0.0031} + 5$$

$\dot{Q}S$ = Flow through shunt.
$\dot{Q}T$ = Flow through lungs.
c = Capillary.
C = Concentration of gas in blood.
$\bar{v}$ = Mixed venous.
PAO_2 = Calculated alveolar oxygen tension.
PaO_2 = Measured value of arterial PO_2.

6. Lung mechanics

— Peak inspiratory flow rate: 300–400 litre/min.
— Peak expiratory flow rate (PEFR):
      450–700 litre/min (male).
      300–500 litre/min (female).
— Compliance:
      Total compliance of lung and chest wall: 0.1 litre/
      cm H_2O.
      Chest wall: 0.2 litre/cm H_2O.
      Lung: 0.2 litre/cm H_2O.
      Airways resistance: 1.6 cm H_2O/litre sec^{-1}.
— Forced expiratory volume in 1 second (FEV_1): 80% of
   vital capacity.
— Maximum ventilatory volume (MVV): 120 litre/min.

7. Alveolar to arterial tension gradient (A − $_a$DO$_2$)

$$PAO_2 = PIO_2 - \frac{PaCO_2}{R},$$

where R is the respiratory quotient (normally 0.8).

$$A - {_a}DO_2 = PAO_2 - PaO_2 \simeq PIO_2 - (PaCO_2 + PaO_2)$$

PAO_2 = Calculated alveolar oxygen tension.
PIO_2 = Tension inspired oxygen.
$PaCO_2$ = Measured value of arterial PCO_2.
PaO_2 = Measured value of arterial PO_2.
Normal adult values at sea level: 5–20 mmHg (0.7–2.7 kPa) breathing air; 25–65 mmHg (3.3 – 8.6 kPa) breathing 100% O_2.

8. Oxygen dissociation curve and causes of shift (Fig. 2.3 p. 48)

Shift to the right
   1.   ↑ temperature.
   2.   ↑ PaO_2
   3.   ↑ red cell 2, 3-DPG.
Shift to the left
   1.   ↓ temperature.
   2.   ↓ $PaCO_2$.
   3.   ↓ red cell 2, 3-DPG.

9. Shunt calculation

To calculate shunt, read off FIO_2% (fractional inspired oxygen concentration) on air/oxygen mixing chart (Fig. 2.4 p. 49). Obtain PaO_2 from arterial blood gas analysis. The percentage shunt can then be determined by using the virtual shunt lines (Fig. 2.5 p. 50).

10. Masks for oxygen therapy

An arterial PO_2 of less than 60 mmHg (8 kPa) at rest is an accepted criterion for the diagnosis of acute hypoxaemic respiratory failure. The aim of controlled oxygen therapy is to raise the arterial PO_2 above this level. Three types of mask are in common usage.

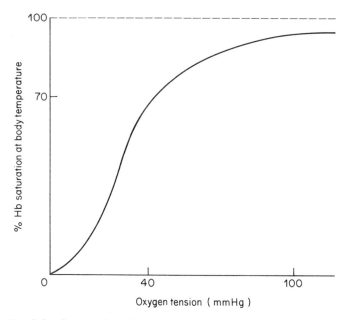

Fig. 2.3   Oxygen dissociation curve.

— Hudson masks
  (When strict use of oxygen concentration is not
  necessary.)

Flow rate (litre/min)	Oxygen in mask
4	40%
6	53%
8	60%
10	67%

— Ventimasks (Vickers Medical)
  These masks produce a fixed FIO_2 by entraining air via
  the venturi principle. There is a choice of five masks
  giving oxygen concentrations of 24%, 28%, 40% and
  60%.

— Continuous positive airways pressure (CPAP) masks
  The principle is to apply, via a tight-fitting facemask, a
  positive airways pressure to spontaneous ventilation.
  Intrapulmonary pressure is increased, opening collapsed
  alveoli and improving oxygenation. A variety of circuits
  which do not require a ventilator are available.

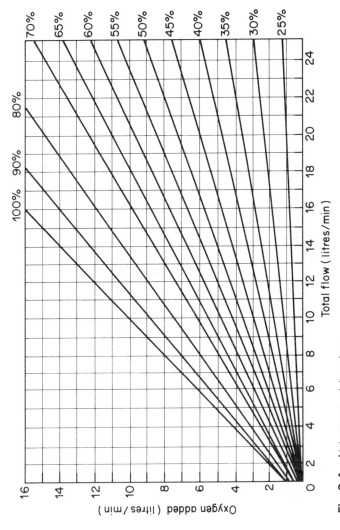

Fig. 2.4 Air/oxygen mixing chart.

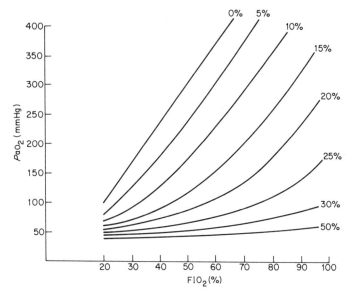

Fig. 2.5   Virtual shunt lines.

Drugs, dosages and infusion regimens

1.   Drugs used in status asthmaticus

Drugs and dosage
(a) β_2 adrenoceptor agonists
* Salbutamol:
  Intravenous bolus
     250 μg.
  Infusion
     5–20 μg/min.
  Nebulized solution
     2.5–10 mg (over 10 min) up to a maximum of
     4-hourly.
  (Nebules = 1 mg/ml in 2.5 ml ampoules and respiratory
  solution = 5 mg/ml which should be diluted in 2 ml
  normal saline for administration.)
* Terbutaline:
  Intravenous bolus
     250–500 μg.

Infusion
   1.5–5 μg/min.
Nebulized solution
   2.0–10 mg up to a maximum of 6-hourly.
   (Respiratory solution = 2.5 mg/ml and 10 mg/ml which
   should be diluted in 2 ml normal saline for
   administration.)
- Rimiterol:
  Nebulized solution
     12.5 mg up to a maximum of 1-hourly (12.5 mg/
     2.5 ml).

(b) Anticholinergic agents
- Ipratropium bromide:
  Nebulized solution
     500 μg–1 mg 6-hourly (250 μg/ml).

(c) Xanthine derivatives
- Aminophylline:
  Intravenous bolus
     5.6 mg/kg over 15 minutes.
  Infusion
     500 μg/kg hour^{-1}.
     ampoules — 10 ml (25 mg/ml) and 2 ml (250 mg/ml).
  Therapeutic range (plasma)
     10–20 μg/ml.
  NB
  —   Extreme care should be taken in patients already
      taking oral theophyllines. In some centres oral
      theophylline administration is regarded as a
      contraindication to systemic therapy.
  —   The effects of aminophylline are potentiated by
      cimetidine and erythromycin.

(d) Steroids
Intravenous hydrocortisone 4 mg/kg 6-hourly overlap-
ping with oral prednisolone at a starting dose of 40–60
mg/day.

2.   Doxapram hydrochloride

Uses
- Chronic respiratory failure.
- Respiratory depression induced by analgesics.

Dosage
Infusion
  500 ml bottle (2 mg/ml) in 5% dextrose at
  0.5–4.0 mg/min.

60 drops/ml	
mg/min	drops/min
0.5	15
1.0	30
1.5	45
2.0	60
2.5	75
3.0	90
3.5	105
4.0	120

NB
— Its action is potentiated by monoamine oxidase
  inhibitors.
— Severe hypertension, coronary artery disease and
  thyrotoxicosis are contraindications.
— Care should be taken in epileptic patients.

3.   Streptokinase

Use
As a thrombolytic agent in venous thrombosis/pulmonary
embolism.

Infusion regimen
• Stop any existing anticoagulant treatment.
• Give hydrocortisone 25 mg oral/i.v. as a single dose and
  continue twice daily during duration of treatment to guard
  against the occasional febrile reaction or anaphylaxis.
• Add 600 000 iu streptokinase (1 vial + 5 ml water for
  injection) to 100 ml 5% dextrose and administer
  intravenously, either centrally or peripherally, over 30
  minutes (this neutralizes any antistreptokinase antibodies).
• Add 600 000 iu streptokinase to 540 ml 5% dextrose and
  administer intravenously over 6 hours (90 ml/hour) and
  repeat for a maximum duration of 72 hours.

• To prevent rethrombosis commence warfarin therapy during the last 24 hours of thrombolytic therapy or start heparin 4 hours after completion.

Control
The thrombin clotting time may be used and should be kept in the range of $\times 2 - \times 4$ the control value.

Complications
— Bleeding:
  ○ Minor — compression.
  ○ Major — stop streptokinase. Administer tranexamic acid, 10 mg/kg, by slow intravenous injection immediately.

Contraindications
— Patients with an increased risk of haemorrhage (e.g. bleeding diathesis, peptic ulceration, previous cerebral haemorrhage).
— Surgery within the previous week.
— Following diagnostic procedures (e.g. lumbar puncture).
— Treatment with streptokinase in the previous 3–6 months (relative contraindication).
— Renal or hepatic impairment.

4. Muscle relaxants

These drugs should only be administered by or in the presence of an anaesthetist, and when full resuscitative facilities are available. These drugs have no sedative action and therefore have only very few indications in ventilated patients.
— Flail chests, where no spontaneous chest movements can be allowed to avoid paradoxical respiration.
— Head injury where movement may precipitate a rise in intracranial pressure.
— Severe hypoxia where optimal gas exchange is critical.
  Muscle relaxants must never be used without sedation.
There are two classes:
— Depolarizing relaxants.
    These mimic the action of acetylcholine at the neuromuscular junction but cause blockade; their

actions are potentiated by anticholinesterases and other depolarizing relaxants.
— Nondepolarizing relaxants.
These cause blockade by competing with acetylcholine at the neuromuscular junction; they are antagonized by anticholinesterases (e.g. neostigmine).

NB
The actions of both classes may be potentiated by antibiotics of the polymixin and aminoglycoside groups. The nondepolarizing relaxants should be avoided in myasthenia.

Depolarizing relaxants

- Suxamethonium
  Dose
    1.0–1.5 mg/kg i.v. bolus.
  Onset
    Almost immediate.
  Duration
    2–5 min.

  NB
  — Contraindicated in:
    ○ Burn victims due to rapid potassium efflux leading to hyperkalaemia.
    ○ Severe liver disease.
    ○ Open eye injuries.
    ○ Malignant hyperpyrexia or positive family history.
    ○ Renal failure.
  — Vagal induced bradycardia following administration.
  — Prolonged apnoea in plasma cholinesterase deficiency.
  — Muscle pain postoperatively.

Nondepolarizing relaxants

- D-tubocurarine
  Dose
    10–15 mg i.v. initially followed by supplements of 5 mg as necessary up to a maximum of 40 mg.
  Onset
    Approximately 3–5 min.
  Duration
    Approximately 40 min.

NB
— Care in patients with renal failure.
— Hypotension and tachycardia secondary to a decrease in peripheral resistance.
— Provokes histamine release.

• Alcuronium
    Dose
        200–250 μg/kg i.v. followed by 1/4 of initial dose.
    Onset
        Approximately 2 min.
    Duration
        20–40 min.

NB
— Hypotension and tachycardia secondary to a decrease in peripheral resistance.
— Care in renal failure.

• Pancuronium
    Unlike the other muscle relaxants, pancuronium causes an increase in pulse rate and blood pressure and therefore is particularly useful in patients with hypotension and cardiac disease (avoid in phaeochromocytoma).
    Dose
        0.05–0.08 mg/kg i.v. for adults with incremental doses of 0.01–0.02 mg/kg as necessary.
    Onset
        Approximately 2 min.
    Duration
        Approximately 40 min (longer acting in the intensive care patient).

NB
Care in renal or hepatic impairment.

• Atracurium
    Useful in patients with hepatic and renal impairment because it is metabolized by nonenzymatic decomposition in the plasma.
    Initial dose
        300–600 μg/kg i.v.
    Incremental doses
        100–200 μg/kg.
    Infusion dose
        300–600 μg/kg hour^{-1}.

Onset
5 min.
Duration
20–40 min.
NB
Causes histamine release.

• Vercuronium
Initial dose
80–100 μg/kg i.v.
Incremental doses
30–50 μg/kg.
Infusion dose
50–80 μg/kg hour^{-1}.
Onset
5 min (more rapid in infants and children).
Duration
20–30 min.
NB
— No cumulative effects.
— Does not cause histamine release.
— Care in renal or hepatic impairment.

Reversal of nondepolarizing agents

Anticholinesterase drugs (e.g. neostigmine) reverse the
effects of the nondepolarizing agents, although they prolong
the action of the depolarizing agent suxamethonium. A
standard regimen is to give:
Atropine 0.6–1.2 mg i.v. (to prevent the muscarinic
actions of neostigmine).
Neostigmine 2.5–5.0 mg i.v. (acts within 1 minute and
lasts for 20–30 min).

5.   Intravenous anaesthetics and sedatives

It is important to remember that the following agents:
  ○ Are only to be used by doctors experienced in their
    use.
  ○ Are not analgesics.
  ○ Must only be administered when full resuscitative
    facilities are available.

1. Intravenous anaesthetic agents

— Thiopentone
    Advantages: ○ Smooth and rapid induction.
                     ○ Reduces intracranial pressure.
    Disadvantages: ○ Slow recovery.
                     ○ Irritant if perivenous injection.
                     ○ Contraindicated in porphyria.
                     ○ Care in renal failure, congestive
                       cardiac failure and
                       hypovolaemia.
    Dosage: Induction
                     100–150 mg (4–6 ml of 2.5%
                     solution) over 15 seconds by
                     intravenous bolus, repeated as
                     necessary after 30 seconds.
                     Infusion
                     0.2–0.4% solution according to
                     patient's response.
— Methohexitone sodium
    Advantages: ○ More rapid recovery.
                     ○ Less irritant than thiopentone.
    Disadvantages: ○ Involuntary movements.
                     ○ Hiccoughs.
                     ○ Tachycardia and hypotension.
    Dosage: Induction
                     50–120 mg over 30 seconds by
                     intravenous bolus or 1–1.5 mg/kg
                     according to patient's response.
                     Maintenance
                     20–40 mg every 4–7 min.
                     Infusion
                     0.1–0.2% solution according to
                     the patient's response.
— Ketamine
    Advantages: ○ Can be administered both
                       intravenously and
                       intramuscularly therefore useful
                       in paediatric anaesthesia.
                     ○ Does not reduce blood pressure.
                     ○ Causes bronchodilatation.
    Disadvantages: ○ Unpredictable rate of onset.
                     ○ Long duration of action.

            ◦ High incidence of hallucinations in adults.
            ◦ Can cause a rise in intracranial and intraocular pressure.
            ◦ Contraindicated in adults with hypertension or history of mental illness.

Dosage: Induction
            (i) 1–4.5 mg/kg over 60 seconds by intravenous bolus,
            (ii) 4–10 mg/kg by deep intramuscular injection.
            Maintenance
            To full induction dose as necessary.

— Etomidate

The use of etomidate for maintenance of sedation is not currently recommended.

Advantages: ◦ Does not produce a tachycardia or hypotension.
            ◦ Useful in combination with opioids (e.g. fentanyl).
            ◦ Rapidly metabolized.

Disadvantages: ◦ Involuntary movements.
            ◦ Pain on infusion and thrombophlebitis.
            ◦ Depresses adrenal function.

Dosage: Induction
            300 μg/kg by slow intravenous injection.
            Maintenance
            100–200 μg/kg.

— Propofol

Advantages: ◦ Short-acting.
            ◦ Very little accumulation (not licensed for long-term therapy).

Disadvantages: ◦ Involuntary movements.
            ◦ Pain on injection.
            ◦ Mild hypotension possible.

Dosage: Induction
            2.0–2.5 mg/kg according to patient's response.

Maintenance
0.1–0.2 mg/kg min^{-1} by
continuous infusion or
increments of 25–50 mg by
repeated bolus injection.

2. Sedatives

Uses
• Sedation and amnesia pre- and intraoperatively.
• Maintenance of sedation in patients in ICU
particularly those on ventilators.
— Midazolam
Advantages: ○ Rapid recovery (cf. diazepam).
Dosage: Slow intravenous injection
2.5–7.5 mg as required.
— Diazepam
Disadvantages: ○ Slow recovery.
○ Pain on
injection/thrombophlebitis
(Diazemuls—emulsion
preparation of diazepam—is less
irritant).
Dosage: Slow intravenous injection
5–10 mg as required.

NB
— Sedatives have no analgesic action.
— Mild hypotension is possible.
— Accumulation occurs with prolonged use.

3. Intravenous opiates

Uses
• Sedation and analgesia pre- and intraoperatively.
• Maintenance of sedation and analgesia in patients in
ICU.

Papaveretum

Dosage
1–10 mg/hour (add 50 mg to 50 ml normal saline) by
intravenous infusion.

Morphine

Dosage
   1–10 mg/hour (add 50 mg to 50 ml normal saline) by intravenous infusion.

Fentanyl

Dosage
   1–10 μg/hour (250 μg (5 × 10 mg ampoules) in 50 ml syringe) by intravenous infusion.

Alfentanil

Initial dosage
   30–50 μg/kg.
Supplemental dosage
   15 μg/kg.
Infusion (children)
   Loading dose of 50–100 μg/kg as a bolus or fast infusion over 10 minutes (3–6 ml/kg hour^{-1}) followed by an infusion of 0.5–1.0 μg/kg min^{-1}.

Buprenorphine

Dosage
   0.3–0.6 mg by slow i.v. injection every 6–8 hours as necessary.
NB
Not recommended for children less than 12 years old.

Meptazinol

Dosage
   50–100 mg by slow i.v. injection every 2–4 hours as necessary.

Phenoperidine

Initial dosage
   2–5 mg (0.1–0.15 mg/kg in children).
Supplemental dosage
   1.0 mg every hour as necessary.

4. Epidural opiates

Diamorphine

Dosage
2.5–5.0 mg (add to 10 ml normal saline) as bolus
injection. Repeat as necessary.
Duration of analgesia
About 6 hours.

Fentanyl

Dosage
50 μg (add to 10 ml normal saline) as bolus injection.
Repeat as necessary.
Duration of analgesia
About 4 hours.

Morphine

Dosage
2–4 mg (available in preservative- and bacteroside-free
solutions of 10 ml) as bolus injection. Repeat as
necessary.
Duration of analgesia
About 12 hours.

NB
— Respiratory depression.
— Nausea and vomiting.
— Urinary retention.
— Dystonia and sedation.
— Itching.

Techniques

1. Intubation

Indications
— To secure, maintain and control a clear airway.
— To enable controlled ventilation.
— To prevent aspiration of stomach contents (e.g. in the
  unconscious overdose who requires a washout, the
  patient with intestinal obstruction, the obstetric
  patient).

— To aspirate secretions from the trachea and main bronchi.

Equipment
— Bag and facemask.
— Appropriate endotracheal tube:
  - Adult male   : 8–9 mm (oral) 7.0–7.5 mm (nasal).
  - Adult female: 7–8 mm (oral) 6.5–7.0 mm (nasal).
— Magill forceps.
— MacIntosh laryngoscope.
— Catheter mount.
— 10 ml syringe.
— Scissors.
— Lubricant (e.g. KY jelly).
— Suction apparatus.

Procedure
• Ensure that all the equipment is in working order and that the ET tube is cut to the required length (twice the distance from the earlobe to the angle of the mouth for an oral tube, and earlobe to the nose for nasal intubation).
• Check on dental state.
• Position the patient's head so that the atlanto-occipital joint is extended:
   Patient supine with head on a pillow.
   Push the patient's crown down with the right hand and rotate the occiput upwards at the same time with the left hand.
   When the jaw falls open the correct position has been achieved (Fig. 2.6).
• Holding the laryngoscope in the left hand, introduce it

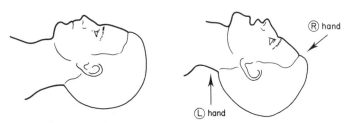

Fig. 2.6   Positioning of head for intubation.

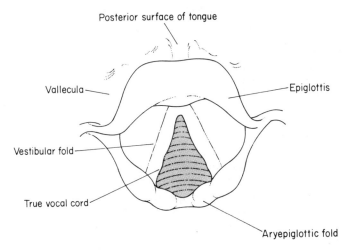

Fig. 2.7 View of larynx at intubation.

to the right of the midline. Displace the tongue to the left and advance the blade until the vallecula is entered anteriorly to the epiglottis (Fig. 2.7).

- Readjust the position of the laryngoscope so that it lies in the midline. Then with a fixed left wrist, move the laryngoscope up and away but do not use the upper teeth as a fulcrum. This should reveal the laryngeal opening as the tongue and epiglottis are moved away from the posterior wall of the pharynx. An assistant can facilitate this procedure by applying external pressure over the larynx. Cricoid pressure also prevents aspiration of stomach contents.
- Introduce the ET tube with the right hand at the right-hand side of the mouth at the level of the premolars so as not to obstruct the view.
- Advance the ET tube towards the larynx and pass it through the cords with a gentle push (difficulty at this stage suggests that the tube is too large).
- Inflate the cuff with air, just sufficient to provide a satisfactory seal, and at the same time attempt to ventilate the lungs from a reservoir bag. Both lungs should be seen to expand. If only one lung inflates, it suggests that the tube has passed down a main bronchus,

usually the right, and therefore needs to be pulled back. Auscultation of the chest following intubation will confirm air entry.
- Secure the ET tube.
- Recheck dental state.

Complications
— Failure to intubate (high risk patients include those with cervical spine pathology, receding jaw and laryngeal tumours).
   ○ Do not persist for too long.
   ○ Ensure adequate ventilation via a face mask.
   ○ Consult a senior colleague.
— Intubation of the oesophagus:
   ○ The chest does not move and no breath sounds are heard on auscultation. 'Gurgling' is heard over the stomach. Remove the tube and reintubate.
— Damage to teeth:
   ○ Retrieve the broken fragments with the forceps.
— Laryngeal oedema:
   ○ Use humidified oxygen and watch the patient carefully. Give dexamethasone 8 mg i.v. Tracheostomy may be necessary.
— 'Sore throat':
   ○ Use care in introducing tube.
   ○ Adequately lubricate the tube.
   ○ Use mild analgesics.
— Tracheal stenosis and laryngeal granulomata.

2. Tracheostomy

Indications
— Upper airway obstruction:
   ○ Acute (e.g. impacted foreign body, laryngeal oedema).
   ○ Chronic (e.g. progressive vocal cord paralysis, tumour invasion).
— Lack of laryngeal reflexes.
— Long term IPPV.
— Following severe injury to the face, jaw, when the airway is in jeopardy.
— In circumstances where oral tracheal intubation is impossible.
— Bronchial toilet.

Equipment
— Appropriate tracheostomy tube and obturator — adult size 28–32 FG.
— Scalpel.
— Dressing pack — gown, gloves, etc.
— Artery forceps and scissors.
— Laryngoscope.
— Magill forceps.
— O_2, suction and anaesthetic machine.
— Humidification apparatus.

Procedure (Fig. 2.8, parts i–iv)
• Anaesthetize the patient (local or general anaesthetic).
• Lie the patient supine and hyperextend the neck.
• Make a vertical incision about 5 cm long sited halfway between the upper border of the sternum and superior border of the larynx.
• Locate the sternomastoid muscles and separate them horizontally identifying the thyroid gland.
• Divide the thyroid isthmus.
• Locate the trachea and make a vertical incision through the 2nd, 3rd and 4th tracheal rings and separate the edges with artery forceps. It may be necessary to excise a little of the anterior surface of the trachea.

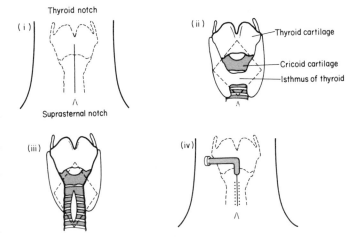

Fig. 2.8 Tracheostomy procedure.

- Introduce the tracheostomy tube and obturator through the incision, and remove the obturator when properly positioned. Inflate the cuff if appropriate.
- Ensure adequate ventilatory efforts occur. If not, apply vigorous suction down the tube and commence artificial ventilation.
- Secure tracheostomy tube (using tapes around neck) and achieve adequate haemostasis. Close wound with interrupted silk or nylon sutures.

Complications
— Displacement of the tube.
— Crusting of secretions due to lack of humidification as the nasopharynx is bypassed.
— Infection.
— Tracheal stenosis/dilatation.
— Sinus and fistula formation.
— Severe haemorrhage as a consequence of erosion of a blood vessel by the tube.

3.   Laryngostomy—emergency

Indication
Unrelieved acute upper airway obstruction when facilities for emergency tracheostomy are not available.

Equipment
— Sharp knife or equivalent.
— Implement to maintain an adequate airway (e.g. barrel of ball point pen).

Procedure
- Lie patient supine.
- Continue/commence cardiopulmonary resuscitation if appropriate.
- Identify the cricothyroid membrane by running a finger down from the laryngeal eminence until the groove between it and the cricoid cartilage is felt (Fig. 2.9).
- Extend the head.
- Incise the skin and insert the knife in the horizontal plane through the cricothyroid membrane by holding the knife

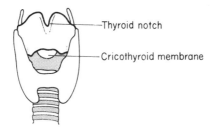

Fig. 2.9 Site for emergency laryngostomy.

at right angles to the skin.
• Rotate the knife through 90° to widen the airway and insert an available implement to maintain the patency of the airway.
• Commence artificial ventilation via the laryngostomy and await help.

4. Artificial ventilation of the lungs

Indications

Inadequate spontaneous ventilation
  Pulmonary pathology:
    With hypoxaemia ($Pa_{O_2} < 60$ mm Hg or 8 kPa with FI_{O_2} of 60%).
    And/or hypercarbia ($Pa_{CO_2} > 60$ mm Hg or 7.5 to 8 kPa).
  — Severe pneumonia.
  — Adult respiratory distress syndrome (ARDS).
  — Pulmonary oedema.
  — Severe asthma.
  — Acute exacerbation of chronic obstructive airways disease.
  Hypoventilation:
  — Central depressants.
  — Neurological damage or disease.
  — Muscle relaxants.
  — Postoperative (opiates/hypnotics).

Elective or therapeutic ventilation
— Raised intracranial pressure.
— Unstable chest with flail segment.
— Postoperative (unfit patient/major surgery).

Ventilator settings

Tidal volume: 10–12 ml/kg. Large tidal volumes may prevent atelectasis but can lead to overinflation of diseased lungs. Start with a low minute volume in the elderly and grossly hypercarbic patients.

Respiratory rate: 10–12/min.

Minute volume: $\simeq$ 100 ml/kg.

Oxygen/air mixture: Aim for Pa_{O_2} of 70–80 mmHg (9.3–10.6 kPa) and Pa_{CO_2} of 30–35 mmHg (4.0–4.7 kPa).
Aim for Pa_{CO_2} of 25–30 mmHg (3.5–4.0 kPa) if hyperventilation is planned. Blood gas values after 1 hour of ventilation will aid further adjustment. If $Pa_{CO_2} < 30$ mmHg and hyperventilation is not required reduce minute volume or add dead space.

Ventilatory pattern: The inspiratory: expiratory ratio should be 1:2.
Inspiratory time
A longer inspiratory time can improve gas exchange by allowing more time for diffusion and prevention of atelectasis.
Expiratory time
In obstructive airways disease expiratory time must be increased to prevent hyperinflation.

Duration of ventilation: A tracheostomy should be considered after 7–10 days of artificial ventilation via an endotracheal tube; earlier if a decision for prolonged ventilation has been made.

Types of ventilators

Flow generators   These have a high generating pressure and flow is unaffected by changes in lung compliance and airways resistance. They do not compensate for leaks in the circuit.

Pressure generators   These have a low generating pressure and flow can be influenced by changes in lung compliance and airways resistance. Leaks are compensated for.

Many modern ventilators are a combination of both types and can be used either as constant flow or constant pressure generators.

Modes of ventilation

Continuous Mechanical Ventilation (CMV)
   Ventilation totally taken over by the machine. Usually intermittent positive pressure ventilation (IPPV).

Positive End Expiratory Pressure (PEEP)
   Intrathoracic pressure remains positive (relative to atmosphere) at the end of each expiration. The functional residual capacity (FRC) is increased, alveolar collapse is prevented, and the distribution of inspired gas is improved. PEEP usually decreases the alveolar to arterial tension gradient $(A-_aDO_2)$ and improves oxygenation. PEEP is particularly useful in cases of high pressure pulmonary oedema as, besides improving oxygenation, it also decreases venous return to the heart and has been said to 'splint' the distended myocardium.
   Adverse effects are mainly due to the resultant increased intrathoracic pressure. They include:
   —   A reduction in cardiac output which may counteract the beneficial effect on oxygenation.
   —   Raised intracranial pressure.
   —   Increased risk of barotrauma.
   —   Reduced renal blood flow and increased aldosterone secretion.

Intermittent Mandatory Ventilation (IMV)
   'Mandatory' tidal volume and rate are preset, but the

patient is allowed to breathe spontaneously in between. The preset rate can be progressively reduced to encourage spontaneous ventilation until the patient can be weaned off the machine completely. In Synchronized IMV (SIMV) the machine synchronizes itself to the patient's efforts to avoid excessive pressure during expiration.

Advantages
— Reduced need for sedation.
— Facilitated weaning process.
— Reduced side-effects of IPPV.

Assisted or Triggered Ventilation
The patients's inspiratory efforts can trigger the machine to deliver a preset tidal volume. The sensitivity of the trigger can usually be altered.

Advantages
— Same as for IMV.

Disadvantages
— Excessive triggering may lead to gross hyperventilation.

○ Mandatory Minute Volume (MMV)
Metered pre-selected minute volume of fresh gas from which the patient breathes as much as he/she is able, the remainder being delivered via a ventilator.

Advantages:
— Same as for IMV.

○ Continuous Positive Airways Pressure (CPAP)
Same principle as PEEP, but the patient breathes spontaneously. Achieved by introducing a resistance to expiration into the circuit.

Advantages:
— Reduces the likelihood of atelectasis and improves gas exchange.
— May be applied via an endotracheal tube or close fitting face mask.
— Alternative to IPPV or during weaning.

○ High Frequency Ventilation
There are three basic techniques:
— High frequency positive pressure ventilation (rate 60/min).

— High frequency jet ventilation (rate 100–200/min)
  delivering gas at high pressure which entrains
  humidified gas via a sidearm.
— High frequency oscillation (5–40 Hz).

Inflation pressures are reduced and ventilation is better
tolerated. It is of particular use in patients with
bronchopleural fistulae and during weaning.

Weaning

Indications to commence weaning
- Normal chest X-ray.
- Haemodynamic and biochemical stability.
- Alveolar to arterial tension gradient (A_a–DO_2) < 300
  mmHg.
- Intact cough reflex.
- Vital capacity of > 15 ml/kg.

Method
The simplest method is to try the patient off the ventilator
for short periods ($\simeq$ 15 minutes) at regular intervals
(hourly/2 hourly) and gradually increase the time.
Humidified oxygen-enriched air (FIO_2 of 70–100%) must be
provided usually via a T-piece during this period.

Alternative methods include the use of the IMV or MMV
mode and progressive reduction in the amount of work done
by the machine.

Successful weaning
- FIO_2 < 40%
- PEEP $\leqslant$ 5 cm of water.
- Negative inspiratory pressure (against occluded airway)
  of −20 cm of H_2O.
- Adequate tidal volume and rate.

Unsuccessful weaning
- Agitation, tachypnoea and cyanosis.
- Rising blood pressure, heart rate.
- Rising $PaCO_2$.

Reventilation during the first night of weaning is often
beneficial.

Complications

Related to the patient
— Hypoxaemia
  ○ Check position of the endotracheal tube.
  ○ Exclude a pneumothorax.
  ○ Decreased FRC and compliance due to ventilation/perfusion mismatch.
— Hypotension
  ○ Decreased venous return due to IPPV.
  ○ Hypovolaemia accentuated by IPPV.
— Increase in airway pressure
  ○ Inadequate sedation/bronchospasm/pulmonary oedema/pneumothorax.

Related to the equipment
— Decrease in airway pressure
  ○ Exclude a leak in the system.
— Increase in airway pressure
  ○ Obstruction of endotracheal tube (mucus plug, malposition, kink, overinflated cuff).

5A. Insertion of a chest drain

Indications
— Emergency — Tension pneumothorax.
  — Thoracic trauma, haemothorax, chylothorax, etc.
— Elective — Pneumothorax.
  — Haemothorax, chylothorax, pyothorax, empyema, etc.

Equipment
— Sterile towels, gown, suture pack, gloves.
— Iodine solution or equivalent.
— 10 ml syringe, 1% lignocaine, No. 11 blade.
— 21G, 19G gauge needles.
— Underwater thoracotomy drainage bottle filled with sterile water to a known level.

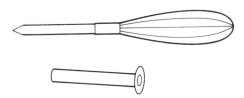

Fig. 2.10   Tudor–Edwards trocar and cannula.

— Sufficient length of red rubber tubing and connectors.
— 2 drain clamps and 1 pair of forceps.
— Chest drain 22F, 26F size (e.g. Argyle, Malecot).
— Tudor–Edwards trocar and cannula (Fig. 2.10).
— Vacuum pump.

Procedure
- Explain the procedure to the patient.
- Select insertion site (Fig. 2.11). For pneumothoraces this can be:
  - Anteriorly in the 2nd intercostal space (ICS) in the midclavicular line.
  - 5th ICS in the anterior axillary line.
  - Posteriorly in the 1st ICS (midway along a line linking the medial border of the spine of the scapula with the vertebral prominence).

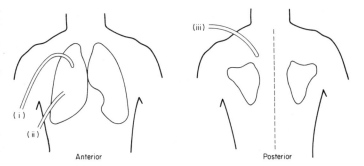

Fig. 2.11   Insertion sites for chest drains. (i) 2nd ICS in midclavicular line. (ii) 5th ICS in anterior axillary line. (iii) posteriorly in 1st ICS.

If fluid or other collections are to be drained, the drain must be inserted at a site relevant to the collection as judged both clinically and radiologically.
- Prepare and towel the proposed entry site.
- Infiltrate the chosen intercostal space with local anaesthetic, taking care to transverse the upper border of the rib with the needle.
- Before removal of the needle check that either air (pneumothorax) or fluid (haemothorax, pyothorax, etc) is aspirated hence confirming correct positioning of the entry site.
- Check that the underwater thoracotomy drainage bottle is appropriately connected (Fig. 2.12) and that the drain is of the correct size (runs freely through Tudor–Edwards trocar).
- Make a 0.5–1 cm skin incision vertically at the entry site.
- Insert one suture at the caudal end of the incision (to secure the drain) and a further suture loosely around the incision (for subsequent closure of the wound).
- Bluntly dissect through the subcutaneous tissue with a pair of forceps.
- *Tudor–Edwards trocar and cannula:*
  Advance the trocar and cannula down the dissection line until the pleural cavity is entered. Firm pressure is required. Remove the trocar and feed the drain through the cannula and then remove the cannula over the drain.
  Argyle drain:
  Advance the drain and introducer down the dissection

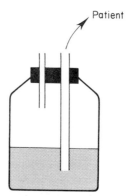

Patient

Fig. 2.12   Underwater thoracotomy drainage bottle.

line until resistance is felt. With a twisting motion (left hand holding the catheter close to the skin and right hand holding the handle of the introducer) carefully increase the pressure applied until the pleural cavity is entered. Then withdraw the introducer a few centimetres, position the drain by angling the introducer and remove the introducer completely.

- Apply two clamps to the proximal end of the drain. Attach the drain to the underwater thoracotomy bottle via the red rubber tubing provided.
- Remove the clamps and confirm that either air or fluid passes into the bottle.
- Suture the drain in position. Apply a dressing around the insertion point and tape it to the skin.
- Perform a chest X-ray to identify the position of the drain and adjust it if necessary.
- For a pneumothorax that fails to expand, it may be necessary to attach a vacuum pump to the short tubing on the underseal bottle and adjust to a suitable pressure (approximately 10–15 cmHg). It is important that a low volume pump does not prevent satisfactory removal of air in the case of a large air leak.
- Record whether the drain is swinging, the pressure of the pump and the volume and nature of drainage at least every 4 hours.
- Finally, check that all staff are aware that the underwater seal bottle must never be placed above the insertion site (not even when the floors are cleaned).

Complications
— Surgical emphysema.
— Perforation of an internal viscus.
— Mediastinal shift leading to pulmonary oedema.
— Haemoptysis from lung puncture.
— Damage to intercostal nerves and arteries.

5B. Removal of a chest drain

Once the lung has fully re-expanded or drainage has ceased, clamp the tube for 24 hours. If the pneumothorax has not recurred or further fluid collected, the drain may be removed and the skin closed with the suture mentioned above.

3 Renal system

Data

1. Routine urine testing

(i) Protein

(a) Boiling test

Principle — Protein is denatured by heat causing a precipitate.

Technique — Filter the urine if turbid. Boil approximately 4–5 ml urine. If a precipitate appears, add 33% acetic acid. Turbidity due to phosphates will disappear; turbidity due to protein will persist.

(b) Albustix

Principle — Protein forms a complex with tetrabromophenol blue to produce a bluish-green colour.

Technique — Dip the strip into the urine and compare immediately with the colour code on the bottle.

False + ve — 1. Infected or stale urine.
2. Detergents (e.g. Cetavlon).

False − ve — 1. Bence-Jones proteinuria.
2. Tubular protein.
3. Addition of acid to the urine as a preservative.

(c) Salicylsulphonic acid test

Principle — The addition of salicylsulphonic acid to protein causes a white precipitate.

Technique — Filter the urine if turbid. Add 2–3 drops of acid to approximately 1 ml of urine.

False + ve — 1. X-ray contrast media.
2. Tolbutamide metabolites.
3. High concentration of uric acid.

False − ve — 1. Stale urine.
2. Bence-Jones proteinuria.
3. Tubular proteinuria.

(ii) Ketones

(a) Acetest

Principle — Acetoacetate or acetone forms a purple complex with nitroprusside in the presence of glycine.

Technique — Place a tablet on clean piece of paper. Add one drop of urine on top of the tablet (serum, plasma or whole blood can also be used). After 30 seconds compare the colour of the tablet with the chart provided.

False + ve — Urine containing bromosulphalein, phenylketones, L-dopa metabolites or 8-hydroxyquinoline.

(b) Ketostix

Principle — This is a strip version of acetest.

Technique — Examine 15 seconds after dipping into the urine.

False + ve — As above.

(c) Gerhardt's Ferric chloride test

Principle — Acetoacetate forms a red-purple colour when combined with 3% ferric chloride.

Technique — Add 3% ferric chloride drop by drop to 5 ml of urine.

False + ve — Salicylates. This can be distinguished from ketones by boiling the urine when acetoacetate will be converted to acetone and the colour will disappear if ketones are present. Salicylates are unaffected.

(d) Rothera's test

Principle — Acetoacetate or acetone form a purple

complex with nitroprusside in the presence of glycine (Ketostix and Acetest are impregnated with the reagents of Rothera's test).

Technique — 5 ml of urine are saturated with a mixture of sodium nitroprusside and ammonium sulphate. 1–2 ml of concentrated ammonia are added and mixed. A purple colour indicates the presence of ketone bodies.

(iii) Bilirubin in urine

Urine containing bilirubin is pigmented and, if the urine is shaken, the froth will be yellow.

(a) Icotest

Principle   — The tablet contains a buffered diazo compound which reacts with bilirubin to form azobilirubin which is coloured.

Technique — A tablet is placed on the pad provided and two drops of urine are added. The test is positive if a purple colour appears after 30 seconds.

False + ve — Chlorpromazine in large doses.

False − ve — Urine containing certain dyes that are coloured in an acid medium (e.g. pyridinium).

(b) Fouchet's test

Principle — Bilirubin, when absorbed onto a barium sulphate precipitate, is detected by its oxidation to green biliverdin with acidified ferric chloride.

Technique — 2.5 ml of barium chloride is added to 10 ml of urine and filtered. Add one drop of ferric chloride to the precipitate and a blue-green colour denotes a positive reaction. A pale blue-grey colour is negative.

(iv) Urobilinogen in urine

(a) Ehrlich's reagent

Principle — Urobilinogen reacts with Ehrlich's reagent to give a pink-red compound in the presence of saturated sodium acetate. This is extractable into organic solvents (e.g. chloroform or amylalcohol).

Technique — Add 2 ml of fresh urine to an equal volume of Ehrlich's reagent. Allow to stand for 5 minutes. Add 4 ml of saturated sodium acetate solution and shake. A red colour denotes the presence of urobilinogen.

False + ve — Porphobilinogen. The colour due to porphobilinogen is not extractable into organic solvents unlike urobilinogen.

(b) Urobilistix

Principle — Urobilistix is the strip version of the above. The colour is not, however, extractable into organic solvents.

Technique — Dip the stix in the urine and read off the colour chart. The colour changes from yellow to intense shades of brown with increasing urobilinogen. *Absence* of urobilinogen cannot be detected with urobilistix.

False + ve — Sulphonamides.

(v) Glycosuria

(a) Clinitest

Principle — The tablet contains copper sulphate, sodium hydroxide, sodium carbonate and citric acid. The blue copper sulphate solution is reduced to red insoluble cuprous oxide in the presence of sugar. Sodium carbonate and citric acid allow rapid solution of the tablet and sodium hydroxide provides heat.

Technique — Mix 5 drops of urine and 10 drops of water. Add the tablet. Wait until boiling ceases. Compare the colour against the chart.

False + ve — Any reducing substance (e.g. lactose, galactose, xylose, ascorbic acid, homogentisic acid, certain drug metabolites).

(b) Clinistix/Labstix/BM-5L/Uristix

Principle — This stix is specific for glucose and utilizes the glucose oxidase reaction. The stix is impregnated with a mixture of glucose oxidase, peroxidase and chromogens.

Technique — Dip the stix in the urine and compare with the colour code.

False + ve — Oxidizing agents (e.g. hydrogen peroxide).
False − ve — Ascorbic acid.

(vi)   Haematuria

(a)   Haemastix

Principle   — Haemoglobin catalyses the oxidation of
orthotolidine present on the reagent strip to
give a blue colour. The test area is much more
sensitive to free haemoglobin than to red
blood cells. Centrifugation of urine will
differentiate between haemoglobinuria and
haematuria.

False + ve — Urine collected in containers contaminated
by oxidizing agents.

False − ve — High urinary ascorbic acid concentration.

2.   Creatinine clearance

- Estimation from plasma creatinine* (inaccurate in liver
disease).

  Males

$$\text{Creatinine clearance (ml/min 70kg}^{-1}) = \frac{88\,(145 - \text{age in years})}{\text{plasma creatinine }(\mu\text{mol/litre})} - 3$$

  Females

$$\text{Creatinine clearance (ml/min 70kg}^{-1}) = \frac{75\,(145 - \text{age in years})}{\text{plasma creatinine }(\mu\text{mol/litre})} - 3$$

- Estimation from 24-hour urine collection and single
plasma sample during collection.

$$\text{Creatinine clearance (ml/min)} = \frac{\text{urinary [creatinine] }(\mu\text{mol/litre}) \times \text{urine volume (ml)}}{\text{plasma [creatinine] }(\mu\text{mol/litre}) \times \text{collection time (min)}}$$

  Ideally, three consecutive estimations should be done.

* Hull, J.H., Hak, L.J., Koch, G.G., Wagin, W.A., Chi, S.L. and
Mattocks, A.M. (1981) Influence of range of renal function and
liver disease on predictability of creatinine clearance. *Clinical
Pharmacology and Therapeutics*, **29**, 516–21.

3. Haemodialyser clearance of a drug

This is of relevance in calculating drug dosages when haemodialyser clearance constitutes a major route of drug elimination.

$$\text{Clearance} = Q \times \frac{Ca - Cv}{Cv}$$

Q = Blood flow through dialyser.
Ca = Arterial inflow drug concentration.
Cv = Venous outflow drug concentration.

4. Drug dosage in impaired renal function*

It is possible to calculate the elimination rate in a patient with renal impairment ($\hat{Q}$) by relating Q_0 (no renal function) to a measure of impaired renal function such as serum creatinine. Values of $\hat{Q}$ are obtainable from published nomograms. In this calculation it is assumed that there is no alteration in absorption, metabolism or distribution of a drug, that no important metabolites are formed and that serum creatinine provides a reasonable reflection of the degree of renal impairment.

— For creatinine clearances $\geqslant$ 50 ml/min — no adjustment.
— For creatinine clearances $\geqslant$ 20 ml/min < 50 ml/min.
   Usual loading dose
   Usual maintenance dose

$$\text{Dosage interval} = \frac{\text{usual time interval}}{\hat{Q}}$$

— For creatinine clearances < 20 ml/min.
   ○ Drugs with $t_{1/2}$ < 6 hours
      Usual loading dose

$$\text{Maintenance dose} = \frac{\text{usual maintenance dose}}{2}$$

      Dosage interval = $t_{1/2}$ of drug
   ○ Drugs with $t_{1/2}$ > 6 hours
      Usual loading dose

$$\text{Maintenance dose} = \frac{\text{usual maintenance dose}}{\hat{Q}}$$

Usual dosage interval

* Bennett, W.M., Singer, I., Golper, T., Feig, D. and Coggins, C.J. (1977) Guidelines for drug therapy in renal failure. *Annals of Internal Medicine*, **86**, 754–83.

5.   Peritoneal dialysis

The frequency of exchange (e.g. 4×2 litre/24 hours), the length of proposed dialysis and the duration of 'dwell' are selected for each individual patient.
The peritoneal dialysis (PD) solution formulation is dependent on the following factors:
—   Osmolality required (determined by the glucose concentration in the dialysate); for example isotonic 1.36% w/v, hypertonic 3.86% w/v.
—   Exchange volume (0.5–2.0 litre).
—   Electrolyte concentration/litre (Na^+, K^+, Mg^{2+}, Ca^{2+}, Cl^-).
—   Lactate/acetate buffer concentration to maintain pH.
Numerous formulations of the above are now available.

6.   Estimation of protein catabolism*

Urea excretion (g/24 hours) $\times 28/60 \times 6/5 = A$.
Proteinuria (Y) $\times 4/25 = B$.
24-hour rise in blood urea (g/litre) $\times$ body weight $\times$ 0.28 = C.
$A + B + C$ = nitrogen loss.

1 mol urea = 60 g.
1 g urea = 100/6 mmol.
Only 28/60 of urea is N_2; molecular weight urea = 60.
1/5 of urinary N_2 loss is non-urea nitrogen.
To convert to protein catabolism multiply by 6.25.
•   This formula is not applicable:
    ○   In patients with renal failure undergoing dialysis.
    ○   If there are large changes in fluid balance.
•   The blood urea correction should only be applied when a positive correction is being made.

- Ignore stool and sweat loss (2–5% of the total daily nitrogen excretion).
- In parenteral nutrition, amino acid leakage into the urine can be considerable when the blood level exceeds the renal threshold. This can be estimated from the urinary samples collected together at the end of the week as total nitrogen loss in grams (from amino acids).

* Lee, H.A. and Hartley, T.F. (1975) A method of determining daily nitrogen requirements. *Postgraduate Medical Journal,* **51**, 441–5.

7. Measurements used to differentiate pre-renal from established renal failure

	Normal	Pre-renal	Renal
Urine osmolality (mOsm/kg)	400–1400	> 400	285–295
Urine/plasma osmolal ratio	> 2:1	> 1.5:1	1.1:1
Urine/plasma urea ratio	> 20:1	> 10:1	< 4:1
Urinary [Na$^+$] (mmol/litre)	< 10	< 10	> 20
Urine specific gravity	1000–1040	1022	1010

Drug dosages in renal failure

The table on pp. 84–88* provides a guideline for drug prescribing in renal failure. For the majority of drugs an initially 'normal' loading dose is appropriate. Dosage supplementation will be necessary for those drugs that are significantly removed by dialysis. (Dialysis refers to haemodialysis, haemofiltration and peritoneal dialysis unless otherwise stated.)

It must be appreciated that the guidelines are not absolute. Plasma levels should be measured whenever possible.

* Bennett, W.M., Muther, R.S., Parker, R.A., Feig, P., Morrison, G., Golper, T.A. and Singer, I. (1980) Drug therapy in renal failure: dosing guidelines for adults. *Annals of Internal Medicine,* **93**, 62–89, 286–325.

Drugs	Major route of excretion	Normal dosage interval (hours)	Dose interval in renal failure (hours) according to glomerular filtration rate (GFR) (ml/min)			Significant removal by dialysis	Notes
			GFR > 50	GFR 10–50	GFR < 10		
Allopurinol	Renal	12–24	12–24	24	24	Yes	
Amikacin	Renal	8–12	12–18	24–36	36–48	Yes	Monitor plasma levels
Amoxycillin	Renal	8	8	8–12	12–16	Yes	
Ampicillin	Renal (hepatic)	6	6	6–12	12–16	Yes	
Amphotericin	Non-renal (hepatic)	24	24	24	36	No	
Aspirin	Renal (hepatic)	4	4	4–6	4–6	Yes	May exacerbate gastric bleeding due to uraemia
Atenolol	Renal	24	Unchanged	48	48–100	Unknown	Dangerous in renal failure
Azlocillin	Renal	8	8	12	12–18	Yes	Sodium salt may precipitate cardiac failure
Benzylpenicillin	Renal	8	8	8–12	12–18	No	Sodium salt may precipitate cardiac failure
Captopril	Renal (hepatic)	8	Unchanged	Reduce dose	Reduce dose	Unknown	May worsen renal failure
Carbamazepine	Hepatic (renal)	12	Unchanged	Unchanged	Unchanged	Unknown	
Cefotaxime	Renal (hepatic)	12	12	12	12	Yes	Reduce dosage by 50% if GFR < 5ml/min
Cefuroxime	Renal	8	8	12	24	Yes	Reduce dosage by 50% if GFR < 5 ml/min
Cephalexin	Renal	6	6	6	6–12	Yes	Reduce dosage by 50% if GFR < 5 ml/min

Chloramphenicol	Hepatic (renal)	6	Unchanged	Unchanged	Unchanged	Yes (haemo) No (peritoneal)	
Chlorpromazine	Hepatic	6–12	Unchanged	Unchanged	Unchanged	No	
Cimetidine	Renal	6–12	12	12	24	Yes	
Codeine/dihydrocodeine	Hepatic (renal)	4	Unchanged	Unchanged	Unchanged	Unknown	
Colchicine	Renal (hepatic)	12	12	12	18–24	No	
Dexamethasone	Hepatic	8	Unchanged	Unchanged	Unchanged	Unknown	Sodium retention
Diamorphine hydrochloride	Hepatic	4	Unchanged	Unchanged	Unchanged	Unknown	
Diazepam	Hepatic (renal, gastro-intestinal)	8	Unchanged	Unchanged	Unchanged	No	
Digoxin	Renal (hepatic)	24	24	72	100	No	Measure plasma levels
Disopyramide	Renal and hepatic	6	6	12–24	24–40	Yes	
Erythromycin	Hepatic	6	Unchanged	Unchanged	Unchanged	No	
Flucloxacillin	Hepatic (renal)	6	Unchanged	Unchanged	Unchanged	No	Sodium salt may precipitate cardiac failure
Flucytosine	Renal	6	6	12–24	24–48	Yes	
Fluorazepam	Gastro-intestinal and renal	24	Unchanged	Unchanged	Avoid	No	Prolonged sedation; avoid in dialysis patients because of danger of encephalopathy
Gentamicin	Renal	8	8–12	12–24	24–48	Yes	Monitor plasma levels

Drugs	Major route of excretion	Normal dosage interval (hours)	Dose interval in renal failure (hours) according to glomerular filtration rate (GFR) (ml/min)			Significant removal by dialysis	Notes
			GFR > 50	GFR 10–50	GFR < 10		
Heparin	Hepatic	4 or continuous infusion	Unchanged	Unchanged	Unchanged	No	
Hydralazine	Hepatic (renal, gastro-intestinal)	12	Unchanged	Unchanged	Unchanged	No	
Hydrocortisone	Hepatic	8	Unchanged	Unchanged	Unchanged	Unknown	Sodium retention
Ibuprofen	Renal	6	6	8	12	Unknown	Sodium retention
Indomethacin	Hepatic (renal)	8	Unchanged	Unchanged	Unchanged	Unknown	Sodium retention
Kanamycin	Renal	8	24	24–72	72–96	Yes	Monitor plasma levels
Labetalol	Hepatic (gastro-intestinal)	8–12	Unchanged	Unchanged	Unchanged	Unknown	
Lignocaine	Hepatic	Bolus or infusion	Unchanged	Unchanged	Unchanged	No	
Lithium carbonate	Renal	8	Unchanged	Avoid	Avoid	Yes	Measure plasma levels
Mefenamic acid	Hepatic	8	Unchanged	Unchanged	Avoid	No	Sodium retention
Methicillin	Renal (hepatic)	4	4	4	8–12	No	Sodium salt may precipitate cardiac failure
Methyldopa	Hepatic and renal	6	Unchanged	9–18	18–24	Yes	
Methylprednisolone	Hepatic	24	Unchanged	Unchanged	Unchanged	Yes	Sodium retention

Drug	Route of elimination					Dialysed	Comments
Metoclopramide	Hepatic	6–12	Unchanged	Unchanged	Unchanged	No	
Metoprolol	Hepatic	12	Unchanged	Unchanged	Unchanged	No	
Metronidazole	Renal and hepatic	8	8	8	8–12	Yes	
Miconazole	Hepatic (renal)	8	Unchanged	Unchanged	Unchanged	No	
Minoxidil	Hepatic	8–12	Unchanged	Unchanged	Unchanged	No	Sodium retention
Morphine	Hepatic	4	Unchanged	Unchanged	Unchanged	Unknown	
Naproxen	Renal	12	12	12	18	Unknown	
Netilmicin	Renal	8	8–12	12–24	24–48	Yes (haemo) Yes (peritoneal)	Monitor plasma levels
Paracetamol	Hepatic	4	4–6	6	8	No	
Phenytoin	Hepatic (renal)	24	Unchanged	Unchanged	Unchanged	No	
Prazosin	Hepatic	8–12	Unchanged	Unchanged	Unchanged	No	
Prednisolone	Hepatic	8	Unchanged	Unchanged	Unchanged	Unknown	Sodium retention
Primidone	Hepatic (renal)	8	8	8–12	12–24	Yes	
Probenecid	Hepatic (renal)	12	12	Avoid	Avoid	Unknown	Ineffective if GFR < 25 ml/min
Prochlorperazine	Hepatic	6–12	Unchanged	Unchanged	Unchanged	No	
Propranolol	Hepatic	6–8	Unchanged	Unchanged	Unchanged	No	
Ranitidine	Renal	12	12	12	Reduce dose	Yes	Safer than cimetidine in renal failure
Rifampicin	Hepatic	24	Unchanged	Unchanged	Unchanged	No	Hepatotoxic; interstitial nephritis reported. Rarely causes renal failure
Salbutamol	Hepatic (renal)	8	Unchanged	Unchanged	Unchanged	Unknown	

Drugs	Major route of excretion	Normal dosage interval (hours)	Dose interval in renal failure (hours) according to glomerular filtration rate (GFR) (ml/min)			Significant removal by dialysis	Notes
			GFR > 50	GFR 10–50	GFR < 10		
Sodium nitroprusside	Non-renal	Intravenous infusion	Unchanged	Unchanged	Unchanged	Yes	
Sodium valproate	Hepatic	24	Unchanged	Unchanged	Unchanged	Unknown	
Sulphonamide/trimethoprim combinations	Hepatic and renal	12	12	18	24	Yes	
Terbutaline	Hepatic (renal)	8	Unchanged	Unchanged	Unchanged	Unknown	
Theophylline	Hepatic (renal)	6–12	Unchanged	Unchanged	Unchanged	Yes	
Ticarcillin	Renal	4–6	6–12	12–24	24–28	Yes	Sodium salt may precipitate cardiac failure
Tobramycin	Renal	8	8–12	12–24	24–48	Yes	Monitor plasma levels
Trimethoprim	Renal	12	12	18	24	Yes	
Warfarin	Hepatic	24	Unchanged	Unchanged	Unchanged	Unknown	

Techniques

1. Peritoneal dialysis catheter insertion

Indications
— Acute/chronic renal failure when:
  ○ Blood urea > 50 mmol/litre, creatinine > 0.88 mmol/litre.
  ○ Development of neurological or cardiac sequelae (e.g. depressed consciousness, pericardial effusion).
  ○ Intractable hyperkalaemia or rapidly rising K^+.
  ○ Fluid overload.
  ○ Intractable acidosis.
  ○ 'Space' required for enteral/peritoneal nutrition.
— Treatment or overdose with dialysable poisons.
— Correction of hypothermia.
— Treatment of acute pancreatitis.
— Diagnostic peritoneal lavage (e.g. peritonitis).

Equipment
— Sterile towels, gown, suture pack, gloves.
— Iodine solution or equivalent.
— 10 ml syringe, 2% lignocaine, No. 15 blade.
— 25G, 21G gauge needles.
— 2 × 30 silk sutures.
— 10 ml syringe containing normal saline + 500 iu heparin.
— Dialysis catheter (e.g. Trocath), PD solution + 'Y' connection set.

Procedure
• Inform the patient of intended procedure.
• Choose appropriate PD solution for commencement of dialysis, and warm solutions to body temperature in an incubator.
• Add 500 iu heparin to each bag of dialysis fluid. K^+ should only be added when the dialysis is running smoothly and initial hyperkalaemia corrected (some commercial solutions contain K^+).
• Ask the patient to empty bladder fully, or catheterize if this is not possible.
• Lie the patient flat, shave and surgically prepare the abdomen.

- Infiltrate down with 2% lignocaine (plain), initially with a 25G needle and then with a 21G needle at the appointed site:
  - One-third of way down a line joining umbilicus and upper border of pubis in midline.
  - Right/left iliac fossa, two-thirds of the way along a line joining the umbilicus and the anterior superior iliac spine (appropriate in patients who have had previous midline surgery).
- Make a small skin incision at proposed entry site with a No. 15 blade and place a 30 silk suture at proximal end of incision in order to secure catheter.
- Examine the Trocath:
  - Ensure stylet is fully inserted into catheter.
  - Note the black markings on the catheter which denote the direction of curvature of the catheter (remove the stylet a few centimetres to demonstrate this).
  - Position the retaining ring over the Trocath so that it lies 2–3 cm from the proximal end.
- Introduce the Trocath through the skin incision until resistance is felt. Two layers need to be penetrated, namely:
  - The abdominal musculature (Linea alba in the midline).
  - The peritoneal cavity.
- Hold the handle of the Trocath in the right hand while controlling the skin and lower end of the catheter in the left hand, and vertically penetrate the abdominal cavity with a twisting motion. Two 'gives' will be felt.
- Withdraw the stylet a few centimetres to prevent damage to the abdominal viscera by the stylet tip and thread the catheter over the stylet in the direction of the pelvis (using the black markers as a guideline) until approximately three-quarters of the catheter has been inserted.
- Remove the stylet and advance the catheter further until approximately 3–4 cm protrudes and the catheter is angled to either left or right iliac fossa.
- Flush the catheter with 10 ml of normal saline containing 500 iu heparin.
- Connect the administration set and run in 0.5–1 litre of dialysis fluid. The fluid should run in easily and when

complete, reverse the flow to ensure satisfactory
drainage. If drainage is not satisfactory:
- ○ The catheter may not have penetrated the peritoneum
  and the fluid may be accumulating in the
  extraperitoneal tissues; the catheter needs to be
  reinserted.
- ○ The catheter may be poorly positioned/blocked with
  abdominal omentum.
- Once satisfactory exchange has been achieved, insert a
  purse-string suture around the catheter and create a seal
  between the surrounding skin and catheter. Do not pull
  the suture too tight, however, as this will cause the skin
  to break down and make leakage inevitable. In some
  instances, particularly in muscular patients, it may be
  appropriate to leave the suture completely loose only to
  be tightened at a later date should any leakage develop.
- Advance the retaining ring down the catheter to the skin
  surface having applied two gauze swabs at right angles to
  each other between the skin and ring and secure by
  bending the ring slightly.
- Apply further swabs over the ring followed by an
  inverted gallipot with a wedge cut out over the catheter
  and cover with waterproof dressings. The gallipot
  prevents kinking of the catheter at the skin/catheter
  interface when the patient moves.
- Trim the catheter so that the connecting piece is flush
  with the gallipot top and commence a formal dialysis
  regimen.

Contraindications (relative)
— Multiple abdominal surgery.
— Bleeding diathesis.
— Severe chronic obstructive airways disease.

Complications

(a) *Blood-staining*
Blood-staining of the dialysate is common, particularly in
the first few cycles, and clears spontaneously. If blood-
staining does not clear:
- Exclude previously undiagnosed bleeding diathesis and
  treat appropriately.

- Monitor vital signs and, if haemorrhage continues, institute appropriate resuscitation and request a surgical opinion.

(b)   Pain
- Check dialysate is warmed to body temperature prior to use.
- Exclude infection of the fluid, which may appear cloudy; culture the dialysate and, if infected, treat with an appropriate antibiotic.
- Add lignocaine 2% to the dialysate.

(c)   Bowel perforation
(A particular risk when the patient has had previous abdominal surgery).
This is recognized by watery diarrhoea containing sugar or by frank faecal staining of the dialysate.
Treatment:
- Remove the catheter.
- Antibiotics.
- Surgical referral.

(d)   Drainage problems
- Check that the administration set is appropriately set.
- Exclude kinks and blockage in the administration set.
- Flush the catheter with heparinized saline.
- Alter the position of the patient.
- If all else fails, reposition the catheter.

(e)   Cardiovascular and respiratory problems
If either the cardiovascular or respiratory system is compromised by the mechanical effect of the dialysate, reduce the volume and increase the frequency of each exchange.

2.   Haemofiltration

Indications
— Rapid removal of fluid in patients with compromised renal function (the fluid removed is comparable to glomerular filtrate with constituents of molecular weight < 10 000 daltons).
   ○ Pulmonary oedema.

- ○ To create 'space' for enteral/parenteral feeding.
- ○ When haemodialysis and peritoneal dialysis are not appropriate (e.g. in compromised haemodynamic states and following abdominal surgery).

Equipment
— A-V access, for example A-V fistula (Brescia—Cimino AV), Quinton—Scribner shunt, Femoral artery/vein cannulation, Femoral artery/subclavian vein cannulation.
— Haemofilter—Amicon 20/Amicon 30 diafilter or equivalent.
— Small bore connection tubing (provided) and two three-way taps.
— 2 × 1 litre normal saline containing 5000 iu/litre and one drip set.
— Heparin infusion pump, 50 ml syringe containing 10 000 iu heparin in 48 ml normal saline and connecting tubing.
— Commercial substitution fluid (where appropriate).
— Three tubing clamps.
— Urinometer.

Procedure
The operating procedure differs slightly according to the make of haemofilter, and it is therefore important to consult the appropriate instructions. In particular, adequate monitoring to include the patient's vital signs and fluid balance and the filter's ultrafiltration rate and volume is essential. The following applies to the Amicon diafilters.
- Ensure suitable AV access is available (see equipment). A blood pump may be necessary if systolic blood pressure $\leqslant 60$ mmHg.
- Remove the selected diafilter from its plastic bag and ensure that no damage has occurred. In general the Amicon 20 diafilter (0.25 m²) is adequate and achieves flows up to 14–15 litres/24 hours.
- Under sterile conditions attach the appropriate tubing to the outlet ports with a three-way tap on the venous and arterial access ends (Fig. 3.1).
- Place the two 1 litre bags of normal saline each containing 5000 i.u. heparin on an elevated drip stand

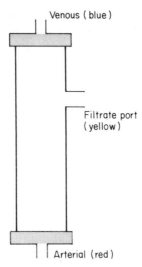

Fig. 3.1 Haemofilter ports.

and attach one 1 litre bag via a standard drip set to the arterial tubing.

- With the arterial end at the bottom, run the first 0.5 litre of normal saline in through the filter as quickly as possible with the filtrate port clamped and the 'free' venous end in an empty sterile bowl.
- Run the second 0.5 litre in with the venous end clamped and the filtrate port open with the filter lying sideways and the filtrate port uppermost. Gently tap the filter to encourage the removal of air from the system.
- Finally, run the second 1 litre of normal saline through, as above, until all the air has been completely removed from the system; then clamp all three tubes.
- Attach the heparin infusion system to the arterial three-way tap and commence the infusion initially at 800 iu/hour and adjust as appropriate (minimum 200 iu/hour).
- Attach the substitution fluid (if indicated) to the venous three-way tap and the ultrafiltration tubing to a urinometer or equivalent.
- Heparinize the patient with a bolus of 1000 i.u. into the venous access, connect the arterial and venous lines appropriately and commence haemofiltration (Fig. 3.2).

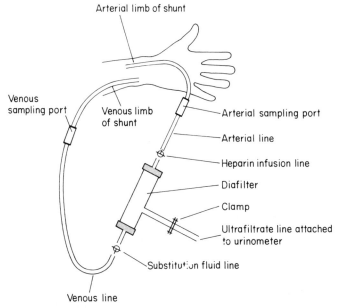

Fig. 3.2 Haemofiltration circuit.

- Place the diafilter upright (arterial end uppermost) in a clamp with the urinometer lying approximately 50 cm below the patient.
- Control the rate of ultrafiltration by a clamp on the filtrate line.
- Once treatment is completed disconnect the arterial line from its access and attach a 500 ml bag of normal saline in its place. Flush the filter until reasonable red cell recovery is achieved.

Absolute contraindications
None

Relative contraindications
— High haematocrit.
— Hyperlipoproteinaemia.
— Poor blood flow.

Complications

(a)   Hypotension
Filtration can be discontinued by clamping off the filtrate line entirely.

(b)   Blood loss/haemorrhage
- Faulty filter (red blood cells in ultrafiltrate).
- Excess anticoagulation.
- Disconnection.

(c)   Haemolysis
This can occur if a pump is used.

(d)   Clotting
Clotting within the pump secondary to:
  ○   Hypotension.
  ○   Inadequate anticoagulation.

(e)   Air embolism

(f)   Hypersensitivity

3.   'Declotting' of an arteriovenous shunt

Equipment
— Sterile towels, gown, gloves.
— Iodine solution or equivalent.
— Two clamps.
— Two 10 ml syringes containing heparinized saline.
— One ampoule urokinase.

Procedure
- Under aseptic conditions apply clamps to both the arterial and venous limbs of the shunt and separate them.
- Attach a heparinized saline syringe to each limb in turn and carefully aspirate. If freeflow does not occur, slowly inject 2–3 ml and then reaspirate.
- If the above is unsuccessful, insert one ampoule of urokinase into the shunt, leave for 1 hour and then repeat aspiration.
- Consider a shuntogram if still unsuccessful.
- Consult a vascular surgeon.

4 Neurology

Data

1. Interpretation of changes in cerebrospinal fluid (CSF) composition (*see* Table on page 98)

NB
— A pleomorphic cerebrospinal fluid (CSF) with a low cell count ($< 1000 \times 10^6$/litre) is common in the early stages of viral meningitis.
— Intracranial hypertension is indicated by CSF pressure > 15-20 mmHg.
— A 'bloody tap' is confirmed by a red/white blood cell ratio of approximately 500:1. 700 red blood cells/mm³ increases the CSF protein content by 1 mg.
— Abacterial meningitis includes:
   ○ Viral meningitis.
   ○ Partially treated bacterial meningitis.
   ○ Meningeal reaction to an intracerebral abscess/granuloma.
   ○ Fungal meningitis.
   ○ Leptospirosis.
   ○ Neoplastic/lymphomatous infiltration of the meninges.
— Ventricular/cisternal CSF has a lower protein concentration than lumbar CSF.

2. Assessment of the unconscious patient

• Control and protect the airway.
• Obtain any available history (e.g. drug overdose, diabetes mellitus).

Interpretation of changes in cerebrospinal fluid (CSF) composition

	Macroscopic appearances	Microscopy	Cells	Protein	Glucose
Normal	Clear	Normal	0.5×10^6/litre lymphocytes	0.1–0.4 g/litre	2.0–3.2 mmol/litre
Bacterial meningitis	Purulent	Organisms on Gram stains of centrifuged deposit	$> 1000 \times 10^6$/litre Predominantly neutrophils	> 0.6 g/litre	< 2.5 mmol/litre
Tuberculous meningitis	Clear (clots on standing)	Alcohol and acid-fast bacilli on auramine stain	$5–1000 \times 10^6$/litre Predominantly lymphocytes	> 1.0 g/litre Up to 6.0 g/litre	< 2.5 mmol/litre
Abacterial meningitis	Clear/milky	Variable	$< 1000 \times 10^6$/litre Predominantly lymphocytes	0.5–1.0 g/litre	Normal

- Perform a full clinical examination and assess the level of consciousness. In particular, check for:
  - Presence of head injury, fractures, bruits.
  - Smell of ketones, acetone, alcohol on the patient's breath.
  - Papilloedema, subhyaloid haemorrhages, diabetic/hypertensive retinopathy.
  - Presence/absence of gag/cough/blink reflexes.
  - Presence/absence of neck stiffness.
  - CSF ottorhoea and rhinorrhoea.
- Investigations:
  - Dextrostix and blood sugar.
  - Rectal temperature (possible hypothermia).
  - Full blood picture.
  - Urea and electrolytes (possible Addison's).
  - Chest X-ray (possible aspiration).
  - Skull X-ray (possible fracture).
  - Urine/blood for toxicology.
  - Lumbar puncture, NB papilloedema.
- Initiate routine nursing care:
  - Ripple mattress/frequent turning.
  - Nasogastric tube/oropharyngeal suction.
  - Paul's tubing/catheter.
  - Eye pads.
  - Physiotherapy.

3. Death certification

Death must always be verified by a medical practitioner, and a death certificate must not be issued by a practitioner unless he/she has been in attendance in the last illness.

Causes of death
The following should be referred to the Coroner's office (via the deceased patient's affairs officer).
— Unnatural death
  - As a result of poisons – accidental, therapeutic, sensitivity, *Salmonella typhimurium*.
  - Within 24 hours of an operation/procedure/anaesthetic.
  - Due to want, exposure or neglect.
  - Due to industrial disease.

— Violent death (e.g. trauma).
— Deaths (sudden) the cause of which are unknown.
— Death of patients admitted unconscious occurring without recovery of consciousness.
— Death in patients in possession of war and disability pension.
— Deaths of persons in legal custody.
— Deaths subject to complaint.
— Death if not natural spontaneous abortion.
— Death from suicide.

4. Brain death (brain-stem death)

Before checking for brain-stem death there must be a positive diagnosis of the cause of irreversible structural brain damage. Any other relevant cause of coma must be excluded (e.g. drug overdosage, primary hypothermia or metabolic and endocrine disturbances).

Diagnosis
The patient is deeply comatose, unresponsive and artificially ventilated.
All brain-stem reflexes are absent:
• The pupils are fixed in diameter and do not respond to light.
• No corneal reflex.
• No oculovestibular reflexes.
• No motor response within the distribution of the cranial nerves.
• No gag reflex or reflex response to bronchial stimulation.
No respiratory effort during a period off the ventilator:
— Blood gas analysis available:
  The $Pa\text{CO}_2$ should be $\geqslant$ 50 mmHg (6.7 kPa).
  ○ Ventilate the patient with 100% O_2 for 10 minutes.
  ○ Disconnect the patient from the ventilator.
  ○ Administer 6 litres/min of O_2 via a catheter inserted down the trachea.
  ○ Observe for 5 minutes. Measure the $Pa\text{CO}_2$.
— Blood gas analysis not available:
  ○ Ventilate the patient with 100% O_2 for 10 minutes.
  ○ Ventilate the patient with 5% CO_2 in 95% O_2 for 5 minutes.
  ○ Disconnect the patient from the ventilator.

- ○ Administer 6 litres/min of O_2 via a catheter inserted down the trachea.
- ○ Observe for 10 minutes.

These tests should be performed and the results recorded on two occasions, ideally separated by at least 2 hours. Two clinicians are necessary, one of consultant status and the other a consultant or senior registrar experienced in the intensive care field.

If the second testing confirms brain-stem death, a certificate should be issued if the coroner is not involved and the relatives should be notified.

5. Organ donation

When a potential organ donor becomes available, four major questions should be asked.

1. Has a state of brain death been diagnosed by a team which is independent of the transplant team?
2. Has permission for organ removal been obtained from:
   — Next of kin.
   — Coroner/coroner's pathologist?
3. Is the donor organ free of disease or damage:
   — Systemic sepsis.
   — Malignancy (other than primary brain tumour).
   — Pre-existing/past history of disease?
     - ○ Renal — e.g. glomerulonephritis, pyelonephritis.
     - ○ Cardiac — e.g. valve disease.
     - ○ Liver — e.g. hepatitis.
     - ○ Corneal — e.g. previous intraocular surgery, polyneuritis (in general, children are less suitable donors).
4. Is the circulation stable?
   — Blood pressure ⎱ administer intravenous fluids,
   — Urine output ⎰ dopamine, mannitol if necessary.
   — Body temperature — maintain temperature > 35°C.

If, after answering the questions above, you think that your patient may be a potential donor then:

5. Advise the appropriate transplant co-ordinator of the above information together with:
   — Age of potential donor.
   — Cause of impending death.

— Blood group, if known.
— Results of latest haematology, chemistry and liver function tests.
— Length of ventilatory support.
— Proposed time of conclusion of brain-stem criteria.
6. If provisionally accepted, take blood samples for:
— Hepatitis B status.
— HIV status.
— ABO, Rh$^+$ and HLA typing.
— 'Other' under the guidance of the transplant unit, and send to the designated laboratory.
7. Follow further instructions as dictated by transplant co-ordinator.
   Close co-operation between respective teams is essential.

Drugs, dosages and infusion regimens

1.   Drugs used in status epilepticus

Drugs and dosage

(a)   Benzodiazepines
• Clonazepam
   Intravenous bolus
      1–2 mg slowly. Repeat if necessary.
• Diazepam
   Intravenous bolus
      0.15–0.25 mg/kg, repeated after 30 minutes if necessary.
   Infusion
      Up to 3.0 mg/kg over 24 hours.
NB
Respiratory depression

(b)   Chlormethiazole
Infusion
   40–100 ml (0.8% solution) at 60–150 drops/min until status controlled; then 10–15 drops/min according to response.
NB
— Respiratory depression.
— Hypotension.

(c)   Phenytoin
Intravenous bolus
   150–250 mg at a rate not exceeding 50 mg/min, followed
   by 100–150 mg 30 minutes later if necessary.

(d)   Paraldehyde
Intramuscular
   5–10 ml.

2.   Drugs used in cerebral oedema

Drugs and dosage

(a)   Mannitol
Infusion
   25% solution at 1–4 mg/kg over 30 minutes 6–hourly.
NB
Care in cardiac failure.

(b)   Dexamethasone
Intravenous bolus
   10 mg (2.5 ml Decadron) followed by 4 mg (1 ml)
   6-hourly for 10 days tapering to 0 mg over the ensuing
   week (higher doses can be used if necessary).
NB
Steroids only seem to be effective when cerebral oedema is
secondary to a focal lesion, particularly malignant and
metastatic disease (vasogenic). They are of no use in
cytotoxic oedema (e.g. water intoxication, severe head
injury). Steroids may be of use in strokes when there is
radiological (e.g. CT) evidence of focal swelling around a
cerebral infarct.

(c)   Pentobarbitone
Intravenous bolus
   20 mg/kg followed by 4 mg/kg 12-hourly.
NB
Monitor plasma levels.

5 Gastrointestinal and metabolic

Physiological data

1. Nitrogen balance

Nitrogen loss (g/24 hours) = (mmol urinary urea/24 hours × 0.028) + 2

(2 = non-urea urinary nitrogen + faecal and skin losses).

This formula needs to be modified in the following circumstances:
— Protein losing enteropathy.
— Excess nitrogen losses in fistulae or effluents.
— A rapidly rising urea.
— Proteinuria.

2. Energy and nitrogen requirements (70 kg man)

	Catabolic	Intermediate	Non-catabolic
Energy requirements (MJ/24 hours)	15–18	11–14	7–9
Energy requirements (kcal/24 hours)	4000	3000	2000
Nitrogen (g/24 hours) for equilibrium	25	14	7.5
Non-protein calories/g nitrogen	135	200	250

Weight loss will occur unless non-protein energy equals the total metabolic expenditure.

Insufficient energy or excess nitrogen results in a rising urea.

A higher energy intake than necessary leads to fat deposition.
If energy intake is moderate or high and insufficient nitrogen is
provided, amino acids pass into muscle, circulatory levels are
low and the liver is deprived of appropriate substrate for
synthesis of albumin and acute phase proteins.

3. Electrolyte, vitamin and trace element requirements for a normal 70 kg man/24 hours

Sodium (mmol)	80 (60–150)
Potassium (mmol)	80 (60–100)
Chloride (mmol)	100 (60–150)
Calcium (mmol)	5–10
Magnesium (mmol)	5–10
Phosphate (mmol)	40
Vitamin A (iu)	4000 (3000–5000)
Vitamin D (iu)	400 (300–500)
Vitamin E (iu)	1.5–2.0
Vitamin K (mg)	0.5–1.5
Vitamin B (μg)	5
Folic acid (mg)	0.4
Thiamine (mg)	10–20
Riboflavin (mg)	2–4
Niacin (mg)	20–40
Pyridoxine (mg)	2–10
Pantothenic acid (mg)	10
Ascorbic acid (mg)	50–200
Manganese (mg)	2–4
Fluoride (mg)	1–2
Copper (mg)	0.5–1.0
Zinc (mg)	2–4
Iron (mg)	1–10
Iodine (μg)	50–200

Practical data

1.   Diabetic states and their differentiation

	Keto-acidosis	Lactic acidosis	Hyper-osmolarity	Hypo-glycaemia
Serum glucose	↑↑↑	Normal to ↑↑	↑↑↑↑	↓
Serum ketones	↑↑↑	Normal to ↑	Normal to ↑	Normal to ↑
pH	↓↓↓	↓↓↓	Normal	Normal
Serum sodium	Normal to ↓	Normal to ↓	Normal to ↓	Normal
Serum urea	↑↑↑	Normal to ↑↑	Normal	Normal
Serum lactate	↑	↑↑↑	Normal	Normal
Extracellular fluid (ECF)	↓↓↓	Normal to ↓↓	↓↓↓	Normal

↑ = increase; ↓ = decrease.

2.   Intravenous vitamin preparations

	Multibionta (10 ml)	Solivito (vial)	Vitlipid (10 ml)
Vitamin A (iu)	10 000		2500
Vitamin D (iu)			120
Vitamin E (iu)	5		
Vitamin K (iu)			150
Vitamin B (μg)		2	
Folic acid (μg)		200	
Thiamine (mg)	50	1.24	
Pyridoxine (mg)	5	2.43	
Ascorbic acid (mg)	500	34	
Riboflavine (mg)	10	1.8	
Nicotinamide (mg)	100	10	
Pantothenic acid (mg)	25	11	
Biotin (μg)		300	
Glycine		100	

3. Constituents of some commonly used parenteral feeding solutions

Solution	Energy (kJ/litre)	Fat (g/litre)	N_2 (g/litre)	$[Na^+]$ (mmol/litre)	$[K^+]$ (mmol/litre)	$[Mg^{2+}]$ (mmol/litre)	$[PO_4^{2-}]$ (mmol/litre)	$[Cl^-]$ (mmol/litre)	[Acetate] (mmol/litre)	$[Ca^{2+}]$ (mmol/litre)
Aminofusin L Forte	1700		15.2	40	30	5		27.5	10	
Intralipid 10%	4600	100								
Intralipid 20%	8400	200								
Perifusin	550		5.0	40	30	5		9	10	
Synthamin 9	1000		9.1	70	60	5	30	70	100	
Synthamin 14 without electrolytes	1600		14.0					34	68	
Synthamin 14	1600		14.0	70	60	5	30	70	140	
Synthamin 17	1900		16.5	70	60	5	30	70	150	
Vamin 9	1000		9.4	50	20	1.5		55	55	2.5
Vamin 9 glucose	2700		9.4	50	20	1.5		55	55	2.5
Vamin 14	1400		13.5	100	50	8		100	135	5
Vamin 14 without electrolytes	1400		13.5							
Vamin 18 with electrolytes	1900		18.0							

4. Alternative parenteral feeding regimens

		1. Central admin	2. Central admin	3. Central admin	4. Central admin	5. Peripheral admin
Vamin 9 glucose	(ml)	1000	1500	1000	1500	1000
Vamin 9	(ml)					10
KCl 15%	(ml)	10	10	10	10	10
Glucose 10%	(ml)	1000	1000			1000
Glucose 20%	(ml)			500	1000	
Glucose 50%	(ml)			500		
Addiphos	(ml)	10	15	10	15	10
Intralipid 20%	(ml)	500	500		500	
Intralipid 10%	(ml)					1000
Nitrogen	(g)	9.4	14.1	9.4	14.1	9.4
Volume	(ml)	2520	3035	2020	3035	3020
Kcals (non-protein)		1800	2000	1800	2400	1400
Fat	(g)	100	100		100	100
Electrolytes Na$^+$	(mmol)	65.0	97.5	65.0	97.5	65.0
K$^+$	(mmol)	55.0	72.5	55.0	72.5	55.0
Ca^{2+}	(mmol)	2.5	3.75	2.5	3.75	2.5
Mg^{2+}	(mmol)	1.5	2.25	1.5	2.25	1.5
PO$_4^{2-}$	(mmol)	27.5	37.5	20.0	37.5	35.0
Cl$^-$	(mmol)	75.0	102.5	75.0	102.5	75.0

5. Electrolyte and trace elements

		Additrace (10 ml)	Addamel (10 ml)	Addiphos (20 ml)
Fe^{3+}	(μmol)	20	50	
Zn^{2+}	(μmol)	100	20	
Mn^{2+}	(μmol)	5	40	
Cu^{2+}	(μmol)	20	5	
Cr^{3+}	(μmol)	0.2		
Se^{4+}	(μmol)	0.4		
Mo^{6+}	(μmol)	0.2		
F^-	(μmol)	50	50	
I^-	(μmol)	1	1	
Ca^{2+}	(mmol)		5	
Mg^{2+}	(mmol)		1.5	
Cl^-	(mmol)		13.3	
Na^+	(mmol)	< 1	< 1	30
PO_4^{2-}	(mmol)			40
K^+	(mmol)	< 1	< 1	30

6. Formulation of a 3 litre parenteral feeding regimen

Synthamin 17 1 litre — daily.
Dextrose 50% 1.5 litre — daily.
Intralipid 10% or 20% — twice weekly.
Addamel (trace elements and electrolytes) — daily.
Solivito (water-soluble vitamins) — alternate days.
Vitlipid (fat-soluble vitamins) — with Intralipid.
Potassium chloride — as required.
Additional electroytes and trace elements — as required.
In addition, intramuscular injections of folic acid 10 mg and hydroxocobalamin 1000 μg are needed once weekly.

This composition provides 3400 calories daily plus an extra 550 to 1000 calories when Intralipid is used. If more calories are required, 20% Intralipid may be given daily. If fewer calories are required, the contents of the bag may be infused over 36–48 hours or Synthamin 9 or 14 may be used.

Generally, the first bag should be administered over 48 hours, the second over 32 hours and thereafter, each bag over 24 hours; thus commence infusions as follows:

Day 1 — 8.00 am.

Day 3 — 8.00 am.
Day 4 — 4.00 pm onwards.
The advantage of commencing the subsequent infusions at
4.00 pm is that the daily electrolyte values will be available
and additions of KCl etc., can be adjusted accordingly. This
regimen provides:

Synthamin 17	1 litre
Dextrose 50%	1.5 litre
Addamel	10 ml
Solivito	1 vial
Nitrogen	16.9 g
Nitrogen calories	400
Dextrose calories	3000
Sodium (mmol)	73
Potassium (mmol)	60
Magnesium (mmol)	6.5
Calcium (mmol)	5
Phosphate (mmol)	30
Chloride (mmol)	83.3
Zinc (μmol)	20
Manganese (μmol)	40
Copper (μmol)	5
Iron (μmol)	50
Fluorine (μmol)	50
Iodine (μmol)	1
Vitamin B_1 (mg)	1.2
Vitamin B_2 (mg)	1.8
Nicotinamide (mg)	10
Vitamin B_6 (mg)	2
Pantothenic acid (mg)	10
Vitamin C (mg)	30
Biotin (mg)	0.3
Folic acid (mg)	0.2
Vitamin B_{12} (μg)	2
Intralipid 10% or 20% with Vitlipid	
Calories	550 or 1000
Volume	0.5 litres
Retinol (μg)	750
Calciferol (μg)	0.3
Phytomenadione (μg)	15

NB
— Solivito does not contain sufficient vitamin B or
vitamin C in a vial.
— Vitlipid may have too much vitamin A.
— B vitamins are degraded by sunlight and therefore
infusions should be shielded by an opaque bag.
— Insulin administration may be necessary to prevent
marked hyperglycaemia either by addition to the
infusion bag or by a peripheral infusion.

Patient monitoring

Daily:
    Full blood count.
    Serum urea and electrolytes.
    Urine urea and electrolytes.
Twice weekly:
    Serum calcium and phosphorus.
    Liver function tests.
    Urine calcium and phosphorus.
    Body weight.
Weekly:
    Serum magnesium.
    Serum zinc.
    Serum iron and total iron binding capacity (TIBC).

Infusion rates in drops per minute
(For standard infusion set)

	2.5 litre	3 litre
24 hours	35	41
32 hours	25	31
48 hours	17	21

7. Constituents of some commonly used enteral feeding solutions (2000ml)

	Volume	Energy	Fat	Protein	Sodium	Potassium	Osmolality
Liquisorb (4 bottles of 500 ml)	2000	8400	80	80	90	90	270 mOsm/litre
Liquisorb MCT (4 bottles of 500 ml)	2000	8400	65	100	90	90	230 mOsm/litre
Triosorbon (5 sachets of 85g)	2000	8400	81	81	85	85	215 mOsm/litre
Peptisorb (4 bottles of 500ml)	2000	8400	22.2	75	120	60	340 mOsm/litre
Clinifeed 400 (4 cans + 125ml water/can)	2000	6700	53.6	60	42	49.4	306 mOsm/litre

8. Formulation of an enteral feeding regimen

Day 1 — 1 can Clinifeed 400 made up to 2 litres (¼ strength).
Day 2 — 2 cans Clinifeed 400 made up to 2 litres (½ strength).
Day 3 — 3 cans Clinifeed 400 made up to 2 litres (¾ strength).
Day 4 — 4 cans Clinifeed 400 made up to 2 litres (full strength).
A glucose polymer, for example Caloreen made up to a 25%
(isotonic) solution, can be added to:
— Increase the calorie intake.
— Increase the non-protein calorie to nitrogen ratio.

Drugs, dosages and infusion regimens

1. Cimetidine

Uses
- Treatment of duodenal and benign gastric ulcers.
- Treatment of oesophageal reflux and stomal ulceration.
- Prophylaxis of gastrointestinal haemorrhage secondary to
  stress ulceration.

Dosage
Intravenous bolus
   200 mg over 2 minutes 4–6-hourly.
Infusion
   ○ Intermittent
          100–200 mg over 2 hours 4–6-hourly, or 400 mg over
          30 minutes to 1 hour via infusion bag (400 mg in
          100 ml) 4–6-hourly.
   ○ Continuous
          50–100 mg/hour.
Intramuscular
   200 mg 4–6-hourly (200 mg/2 ml ampoule).
NB
— Reduce the dose in patients with renal impairment.
— It potentiates the effect of oral anticoagulants,
   β-blockers, theophylline and phenytoin.

2. Ranitidine

Uses
(*See* cimetidine).

Dosage
Intravenous bolus
  50 mg every 6–8 hours.
Infusion
  25 mg/hour for 2 hours, 6–8-hourly as necessary.
NB
— Preferred to cimetidine in patients on certain interacting drugs (oral anticoagulants, β-blockers, theophylline and phenytoin).
— Lacks the mild androgenic effects seen with cimetidine.

3. Vasopressin

Use
Emergency reduction of portal venous pressure in variceal haemorrhage.

Dosage
Intravenous bolus
  20 units in 100 ml 5% dextrose over 15 minutes.
Infusion
  0.2–0.4 units/min i.v. for a maximum of 2 hours.
Sublingual nitroglycerin can be used in addition:
— To reduce the cardiac side-effects.
— To enhance the reduction in portal pressure.
NB Vasopressin can cause:
— Facial pallor.
— Bowel evacuation.
— Abdominal pain.
— Coronary vasoconstriction.
— Peripheral gangrene.

4. Terlipressin

(A synthetic analogue of vasopressin with reduced side-effects).

Use
(*See* vasopressin)

Dosage
Intravenous bolus
  2 mg 6-hourly, up to a maximum of 72 hours.

5. Lactulose

Use
Portal–systemic encephalopathy.

Dosage
Oral
   6–10 5 ml spoonfuls t.i.d. initially. Adjust to produce 2–3
   soft stools/day.

6. Neomycin

Use
Portal–systemic encephalopathy.

Dosage
Oral
   1 g 4-hourly.
NB
—   Reduce dosage in renal impairment.
—   Avoid concurrent administration of other
     ototoxic/nephrotoxic drugs.

Techniques

1. Insertion of a Sengstaken–Blakemore tube

Indication
Control of variceal haemorrhage.

Equipment
—   Sengstaken–Blakemore tube.
—   Local anaesthetic spray.
—   Nasogastric tube.

Procedure
•   Inform the patient and try to give an indication of how
     long the tube may be in place.
•   Place the patient in the left lateral decubitus position and
     spray the mouth and pharynx with local anaesthetic.
•   Aspirate the pharynx, oesophagus and stomach via a
     nasogastric tube.

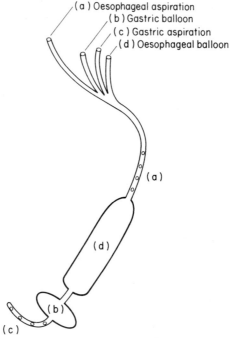

Fig. 5.1 Components of a Sengstaken–Blakemore tube.

- Check the patency and adequate function of the various channels (Fig. 5.1):
  - Oesophageal aspiration.
  - Gastric balloon.
  - Gastric aspiration.
  - Oesophageal balloon.
- Pass the tube via the mouth whilst continuously aspirating through (a). A guide wire in channel (c) may be required to facilitate introduction of the tube.
- When inserted to the required distance, flush (c) with air and auscultate over the epigastric area to check that the stomach has been entered.
- Inflate balloon (b) with 300 ml air (alternatively normal saline mixed with hypaque can be used).
- Withdraw the tube until the gastric balloon creates a traction force on the cardio-oesophageal junction.

- Commence regular aspiration through lines (a) and (c).
- Inflate the balloon (d) with 100 ml air to a pressure of 30–40 mmHg.
- Elevate the head of the bed slightly (20 cm) and secure the tube in position with appropriate traction by taping it securely to the side of the face.
- Insert an oropharyngeal airway if necessary to prevent the patient biting on the tube.
- Check that the traction is adequate every 2 hours and measure the oesophageal pressure every 4 hours with the aid of a manometer.
- After 24 hours release the traction and deflate the oesophageal balloon leaving the gastric balloon *in situ*. If further bleeding occurs the oesophageal balloon can be inflated for a further 12 hours.
- Beyond this time (and ideally much sooner) a definitive procedure must be performed if bleeding continues.

Complications
— Respiratory distress secondary to migration of the oesophageal balloon into the hypopharynx.
— Aspiration.
— Oesophageal/gastric ulceration and haemorrhage.

2. Insertion of a fine-bore feeding tube

Indications
— Patients unable or lacking the desire to eat:
   ○ Elderly.
   ○ Intercurrent illness.
   ○ Altered conscious level.
   ○ Oesophageal carcinoma.
— Catabolic patients not ingesting enough food.
— Malabsorption states.

Procedure
- Inform the patient.
- Empty the stomach with a standard nasogastric tube and ensure, when indicated, that the stomach is emptying properly by introducing a feeding regimen gradually, viz:
   ○ 60 ml/hour water aspirating 4-hourly for 24 hours.
   ○ ½ strength feed for next 24 hours followed by full strength thereafter, then aspirating intermittently.

This is not necessary if gastric emptying is known to be normal.
- Remove the nasogastric tube and replace it with a fine-bore nasogastric tube.
  - Lubricate the guide wire and introduce it into the tube.
  - Pass the wire and tube via the nose into the oesophagus and stomach.
  - Withdraw the wire and attach the proximal end of the tube to the patient's nose and forehead.
- Perform an X-ray or auscultate over the epigastrium whilst syringing air down the tube to check the position of its distal end (the bronchi can be intubated).
- Attach the appropriate drip system to the male luer on the fine-bore tube.

Complications
— Insertion into bronchial tree.
— Blockage:
  - Flush with normal saline.
  - Replace.
— Aspiration due to displacement of the tube or regurgitation of the feed.
— Oesophagitis/ulceration.
— Complications of the feed (e.g. diarrhoea, hyperosmolar states).

6 Toxicology

Data

1. Interpretation of toxicology results

The following data are given by kind permission of Dr B. Widdop, Consultant Biochemist of the Poisons Unit of New Cross Hospital, London, UK.

The concentrations are approximate. Age, previous drug exposure and concomitant clinical disease are not accounted for. Particular care should be taken in cases of multiple drug ingestion. All drug concentrations are expressed as mg/litre of plasma unless otherwise stated.

	Normal concentrations — less than	Concentration associated with severe toxicity
Alcohols		
Ethanol	—	3.00 g/litre
Methanol	—	0.20 g/litre
Analgesics		
Narcotics		
Dextroproproxyphene	0.3	1
Codeine	0.1	1
Methadone	0.1	1
Morphine	0.05	0.3
Pentazocine	0.2	1
Pethidine	0.5	2
Non-narcotics		
Paracetamol	20 (0.13 mmol/litre)	200 (1.32 mmol/litre) 4 hours postingestion 70 (0.46 mmol/litre) 12 hours postingestion
Salicylate	250	600

	Normal concentrations — less than	Concentration associated with severe toxicity
Anticonvulsants		
Carbamazepine	10	50
Clonazepam	0.05	1
Ethosuximide	80	—
Phenytoin	20	40
Primidone	12	100
Sulthiame	12	30
Sodium valproate	80	—
Antidepressants		
Amitriptyline (plus nortriptyline)	0.2	1
Clomipramine (plus norclomipramine)	0.5	1
Dothiepin (plus nordothiepin)	0.3	1
Doxepin (plus nordoxepin)	0.2	1
Imipramine (plus desipramine)	0.3	1
Mianserin	0.1	0.5
Nortriptyline	0.15	1
Protriptyline	0.2	1
Trimipramine (plus nortrimipramine)	0.3	1
Antihypertensives		
Oxprenolol	0.2	2
Propranolol	0.1	2
Anti-inflammatories		
Oxyphenylbutazone	100	200
Phenylbutazone	100	200
Antimalarials		
Chloroquine	0.2	1
Quinine/quinidine	5	10
Cardioactive		
Digoxin	2 μg/litre	4 μg/litre
Disopyramide	3	8
Lignocaine	5	8
Mexiletine	1.5	3
Procainamide	8	16
Quinidine	5	10

	Normal concentrations — less than	Concentration associated with severe toxicity
Hypnotics		
Barbiturates		
Butobarbitone	10	80
Barbitone	15	100
Phenobarbitone	30	100
other barbiturates	5	40
Non-barbiturates		
Chlormethiazole	2	10 (oral dose)
Ethchlorvynol	20	100
Glutethimide	4	30
Meprobamate	10	40
Methaqualone	4	20
Trichloroethanol	10	50
Stimulants		
Amphetamine	0.1	0.5
Methylamphetamine	0.05	0.3
Fenfluramine	0.2	0.5
Cocaine	0.3	3.0
Tranquillizers		
Benzodiazepines		
Chloridiazepoxide	1	5
Diazepam	1	5
Nordiazepam	1.5	5
Flunitrazepam	0.05	—
Desalkylflurazepam	0.15	0.5
Lorazepam	0.2	—
Nitrazepam	0.2	2
Oxazepam	1	5
Phenothiazines		
Chlorpromazine	0.1	1
Thioridazine	1	5
Miscellaneous		
Bromide	14	200
Dinitro-orthocresol	5	50
Ethylene glycol	—	500
Haloperidol	0.1	0.5
Iron Children	1.8 (34 μmol/litre)	5 (90 μmol/litre)
Adults	1.8 (34 μmol/litre)	8 (145 μmol/litre)
Orphenadrine	0.2	2
Paraquat	—	0.5 (6 hours postingestion) 0.25 (12 hours postingestion)
Theophylline	20	40

Drugs and dosage

Activated charcoal

Dosage — 1 part poison to 10 parts charcoal.
(Medicoal, 5 g sachet; Charcoal powder, 50 g).
— 10 g in 100 ml water to a maximum of 50 g is a
usual dose.

Syrup of ipecacuanha

Dosage — 30 ml suspended in water/fruit juice (10–15 ml
for children).
Vomiting will occur within 30 minutes.

NB
— Do not give if conscious level of patient is impaired, as
aspiration of vomit may occur.
— Prolonged vomiting can lead to gastric rupture,
Mallory–Weiss tears, pneumomediastinum and
pneumoperitoneum.
— Delayed adverse effects on the myocardium described.

Poisoning

Agents responsible for poisoning are listed in alphabetical
order. In each case specific management is given in note
form. Intensive supportive treatment is the cornerstone of
management and can include:
— Respiratory
Cardiovascular } support.
Renal
— Temperature assessment and regulation.
— Decontamination of skin, mucous membranes and eyes.
— Gastric lavage/emesis.
— Administration of absorbents when necessary.

Arsenic

1. Dimercaprol 4 mg/kg by deep intramuscular injection
every 4 hours for 48 hours followed by 3 mg/kg b.d. for
a maximum of 8 days.
2. Haemodialysis/peritoneal dialysis if anuria or oliguria.

Barbiturates

Long-acting	: Barbitone.
	Phenobarbitone.
Medium-acting:	Butobarbitone.
	Allobarbitone.
	Amylobarbitone.

1. Forced alkaline diuresis if plasma concentration is:
   Phenobarbitone ⎤
   Butobarbitone ⎬ > 100 mg/litre.
   Barbitone   ⎦
2. Haemoperfusion or haemodialysis if plasma concentration > 150 mg/litre.

β-blockers

1. Continuous ECG monitoring.
2. Atropine 0.3–0.6 mg i.v. repeated as necessary.
3. Isoprenaline 1–3 mg i.v.
4. Glucagon 5–10 mg i.v. followed by an infusion at 1.5 mg/hour.
5. Salbutamol nebulizer/i.v. for bronchospasm.

Bromides

1. Saline diuresis ± frusemide.
2. ± haemodialysis.

Carbon monoxide

1. Remove patient from contaminated atmosphere.
2. 100% O_2 ± ventilation.
3. 95% O_2 ± 5% CO_2 (as a respiratory stimulant)—controversial.
4. Hyperbaric O_2 should be considered for:
   ○ Patients who are or have been unconscious.
   ○ Patients with neurological or psychiatric signs or more than a mild headache.
   ○ Patients with cardiac complications.
   ○ Patients with COHb levels greater than 40%.
   ○ Pregnant women.

Chlorates

1. Methylene blue 1% by slow intravenous injection.
2. Haemodialysis/peritoneal dialysis if anuria/oliguria.

Corrosives

1. Gastric lavage contraindicated.
2. Early examination of the mouth and pharynx followed by endoscopy.
3. Broad-spectrum antibiotics.
4. ± parenteral feeding.
5. Surgical assessment.

Cyanide

Inhalation
1. Remove patient from contaminated atmosphere.
2. 100% O_2.
3. Dicobalt edetate 300–600 mg i.v. over 1 minute + hydroxocobalamin 4 g i.v.

Ingestion
1. Gastric lavage with 300 ml 25% sodium thiosulphate.
2. Dicobalt edetate 300–600 mg i.v. over 1 minute + hydroxocobalamin 4 g i.v.

Digitalis

Therapeutic range of digoxin: 1.3–2.5 nmol/litre.
1. Caution with gastric lavage because vagal stimulus exacerbates pre-existing bradycardia. It is wise to give atropine 0.3–0.6 mg i.v. before the procedure if bradycardia significant.
2. Consider oral cholestyramine/charcoal following lavage to interrupt the enterohepatic pathway if digitoxin overdose.
3. Hyperkalaemia: intravenous aldosterone antagonists (not glucose and insulin).
4. Hypokalaemia: intravenous infusion 20–40 mmol KCl.
5. Lignocaine 100 mg i.v./intravenous phenytoin for ventricular ectopic beats.
6. Demand pacing.
7. β antagonists (e.g. practolol) for tachycardia if pacing wire *in situ*.

8. Digoxin specific Fab fragments (test dose first because of anaphylaxis).
9. Amiodarone intravenously*.

Distalgesic

1. Respiratory depression: intravenous naloxone.
2. Paracetamol: (*see* page 127).

Ethanol

1. Treat hypoglycaemia with intravenous glucose.
2. Fructose (500 ml 4% solution) 200 g i.v. over 30 min.
3. Naloxone intravenously (controversial).

Ethylene glycol

1. Treat metabolic acidosis with intravenous $NaHCO_3$.
2. Give ethylalcohol (50%) 1 ml/kg p.o. followed by 0.5 ml/kg over 2 hours to maintain a blood ethanol of 1000–2000 mg/litre.
3. Early haemodialysis.

Glutethimide

1. Gastric lavage with castor oil and water in equal proportions; leave 50 ml castor oil in the stomach.
2. Haemoperfusion if plasma concentration > 40 mg/litre.

Iron

1. Gastric lavage with desferrioxamine 2 g/litre. Desferrioxamine 10 g in 50 ml water should be left in the stomach at completion.
2. Desferrioxamine 2 g in 100 ml i.m. repeated 12-hourly followed by an intravenous infusion of 15 mg/kg hour^{-1} to a maximum of 80 mg/kg in 24 hours.
3. Haemodialysis/peritoneal dialysis if anuria/oliguria.

Lead

Normal levels < 1.5 μmol/litre.
1. Calcium disodium edetate 50–75 mg/kg i.v. daily for 5 days (each 2 g should be diluted in 250 ml normal saline).
2. In severe overdosage, add dimercaprol 2.5–5.0 mg/kg

4-hourly by deep intramuscular injection for 24 hours.
3.   In mild overdosage, penicillamine 250 mg–2 g/day p.o. until lead levels satisfactory.

Lithium

Therapeutic range: 1–2 nmol/litre.
1.   Forced alkaline diuresis (watch [Na$^+$] and [K$^+$] carefully) – controversial.
2.   Chlorothiazide 0.5–1.0 g/day for diabetes insipidus.
3.   Clonazepam or diazepam intravenous for convulsions.
4.   Peritoneal dialysis or haemodialysis if plasma concentration > 5 nmol/litre.

Meprobamate

1.   Haemoperfusion if plasma concentration > 100 mg/litre.

Mercury

1.   Gastric lavage with 250 ml 5% solution of sodium formaldehyde sulphoxylate.
     100 ml of solution should be left in the stomach at completion.
2.   Dimercaprol (*see* arsenic on page 122).
3.   Haemodialysis or peritoneal dialysis if anuria or oliguria.

Methanol

1.   Treat metabolic acidosis with intravenous NaHCO$_3$.
2.   Give ethylalcohol (50%) 1 ml/kg p.o. followed by 0.5 ml/kg over 2 hours to maintain blood ethanol of 1000–2000 mg/litre.
3.   Haemodialysis if plasma concentration > 0.5 g/litre or signs of mental/visual complications.
4.   Peritoneal dialysis (only if haemodialysis not available).

Methaqualone

1.   Haemoperfusion if plasma concentration > 40 mg/litre.

Monoamine oxidase inhibitors

1.   Avoid sympathomimetics.

2. Clonazepam/diazepam intravenously for convulsions.
3. Chlorpromazine intramuscularly/intravenously for agitation.
4. Haemodialysis for severe overdose.

Narcotics

(Including d-propoxyphene, methadone, dipipanone, diphenoxylate and dihydrocodeine but not buprenorphine).

1. Naloxone 1.2–1.6 mg i.v. and repeated as necessary at 2–3 minute intervals or by infusion (2 mg naloxone in 500 ml 5% dextrose/normal saline) at a rate according to response.

Organophosphorus compounds

1. Decontaminate skin and eyes as soon as possible.
2. Atropine intravenously until full atropinization is achieved (doses up to 1.5 g have been given).
3. Pralidoxime 1 g i.v. followed by up to three further doses over the next few hours (may precipitate convulsions).

Paracetamol

1. Treatment with acetylcysteine (Parvolex) according to protocol (*see* Figs. 6.1, 6.2, pages 129, 130).
2. Alternatively, oral methionine 2.5 g initially followed by three further doses of 2.5 g every 4 hours according to plasma paracetamol concentration.
3. ± haemoperfusion.

NB
Flushing, wheeze and hypotension described during acetylcysteine infusion. Treat with intravenous injection of an antihistamine (H_1 blocker). Stop infusion and recommence at a slower rate.

Acetylcysteine dosage guide†

1st dose = 150 mg/kg acetylcysteine infused in 200 ml 5% dextrose over 15 minutes

†Published with kind permission of Dr L.F. Prescott, University Department of Clinical Pharmacology. The Royal Infirmary, Edinburgh, UK, and Duncan, Flockhart and Co Ltd., UK.

2nd dose = 50 mg/kg in 500 ml 5% dextrose over 4 hours
3rd dose = 100 mg/kg in 1 litre 5% dextrose over the next
          16 hours

Body weight (kg)	Dose	Acetylcysteine Dose (ml)	Acetylcysteine No. of ampoules	Body weight (kg)	Dose	Acetylcysteine Dose (ml)	Acetylcysteine No. of ampoules
40	1st	30	3.0	68	1st	51	5.1
	2nd	10	1.0		2nd	17	1.7
	3rd	20	2.0		3rd	34	3.4
44	1st	33	3.3	72	1st	54	5.4
	2nd	11	1.1		2nd	18	1.8
	3rd	22	2.2		3rd	36	3.6
48	1st	36	3.6	76	1st	57	5.7
	2nd	12	1.2		2nd	19	1.9
	3rd	24	2.4		3rd	38	3.8
52	1st	39	3.9	80	1st	60	6.0
	2nd	13	1.3		2nd	20	2.0
	3rd	26	2.6		3rd	40	4.0
56	1st	42	4.2	84	1st	63	6.3
	2nd	14	1.4		2nd	21	2.1
	3rd	28	2.8		3rd	42	4.2
60	1st	45	4.5	88	1st	66	6.6
	2nd	15	1.5		2nd	22	2.2
	3rd	30	3.0		3rd	44	4.4
64	1st	48	4.8	92	1st	69	6.9
	2nd	16	1.6		2nd	23	2.3
	3rd	32	3.2		3rd	46	4.6

Paraquat

1. Decontaminate skin and eyes as soon as possible.
2. Emesis.
3. Careful gastric lavage if emesis unsuccessful, leaving 250 ml absorbent containing 30% Fuller's earth + 5% magnesium sulphate in the stomach.
4. Follow by oral administration of 30% Fuller's earth suspension 200–500 ml 2-hourly for 24 hours and then 6-hourly for 24 hours.
5. Avoid O_2 therapy if possible.
6. ± haemoperfusion.

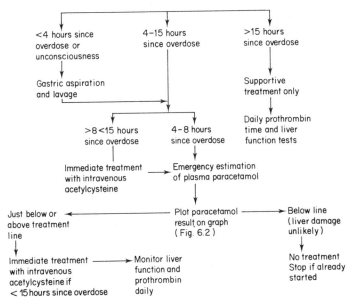

Fig. 6.1 Management of paracetamol overdose in adults with acetylcysteine.†

1. If it is reasonably certain that < 7.5 g have been taken, liver damage is unlikely and no further treatment is necessary.
2. If the time of ingestion is not known (e.g. in the unconscious patient) treatment with acetylcysteine should be started immediately.
3. Results of plasma paracetamol estimation cannot be interpreted < 4 hours after ingestion of the overdose.
4. Acetylcysteine is very effective when given up to 8 hours after overdose. The effect falls off slowly between 8 and 10 hours, more rapidly after 10 hours and increasingly between 12 and 15 hours. It is ineffective after 15 hours and may then be associated with harmful effects.

†Published with kind permission of Dr L.F. Prescott, University Department of Clinical Pharmacology. The Royal Infirmary, Edinburgh, UK, and Duncan, Flockhart and Co Ltd., UK.

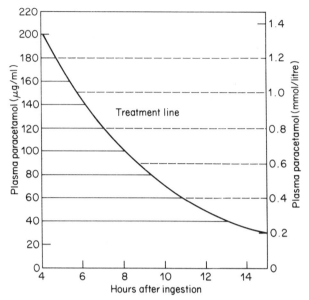

Fig. 6.2   Graph of plasma paracetamol concentration/hours after ingestion.†
Paracetamol concentrations in relation to time after overdosage as a guide to prognosis. Acetylcysteine (Parvolex) is indicated in patients with values just below or above the treatment line.
(Adapted from Prescott, L.F. (1978) *Health Bulletin*, **4**, 204.)

Petroleum

1. Gastric lavage contraindicated unless endotracheal tube *in situ*.
2. 250 ml liquid paraffin orally.

Phenothiazines

1. Dyskinesia
       Procyclidine HCl 5–10 mg i.v.
2. Malignant hyperthermia
       Dantrolene 1 mg/kg i.v., repeated at 5–10 minute intervals to a maximum of 10 mg/kg.

†Published with kind permission of Dr L.F. Prescott, University Department of Clinical Pharmacology. The Royal Infirmary, Edinburgh, UK, and Duncan, Flockhart and Co Ltd., UK.

Phosphorus

1. Gastric lavage in 0.1% copper sulphate solution.
2. Decontaminate burns in 1% copper sulphate solution.
3. ± exchange transfusion.

Quinine/quinidine

1. Continuous ECG monitoring.
2. Stellate ganglion block—visual impairment.
3. Haemolysis—intravenous steroids.
4. QRS widening—infusion of molar lactate.
5. Forced acid diuresis.

Salicylates

1. Gastric lavage ≤ 12 hours.
2. High fluid intake + alkaline urine (*see* forced alkaline diuresis, p. 133).
3. Correction of hypokalaemia.
4. Hypoglycaemia - intravenous glucose.
5. Hypoprothrombinaemia - intravenous vitamin K.
6. Forced alkaline diuresis if plasma concentration > 500 mg/litre.
7. Haemodialysis/haemoperfusion if plasma concentration > 750 mg/litre or 500 mg/litre with superimposed renal impairment.

Theophylline

1. Correct hypokalaemia.
2. Haemoperfusion if theophylline plasma concentration > 60 mg/litre.

Tricyclic antidepressants

1. Gastric lavage ≤ 12 hours.
2. Continuous ECG monitoring.
3. Clonazepam/diazepam for convulsions.
4. Physostigmine 2–4 mg i.v. for anticholinergic effects (tachycardia, confusion) - controversial.

* Maheswaran, R., Bramble, M.G. and Hardisty, C.A. (1983). Massive digoxin overdose: Successful treatment with intravenous amiodarone. *British Medical Journal,* **287**, 392-3.

Techniques

1.   Gastric lavage

Indications
— Overdose in an unconscious patient when:
  ○ Poison or poisons are unknown.
  ○ Time of ingestion is unknown.
— Within 4 hours of ingestion of a significant amount of poison(s) or within 12 hours in salicylates or other poisons that delay gastric emptying.

Equipment
— Wide bore (30 gauge) soft rubber tube (e.g. Jacques 30).
— Funnel.

Procedure
• Assess conscious level of the patient and absence/presence of a cough/gag reflex. Request a cuffed endotracheal tube insertion if appropriate.
• Obtain consent if possible.
• Place the patient on a tilt table in the semiprone position with the patient's head over the side at approximately 30°.
• Insert an appropriate soft rubber tube into the stomach and aspirate (gastro-oesophageal junction is approximately 40 cm from the mouth).
• Once aspiration is complete (check that tube is not in the trachea), repeatedly wash approximately 500 ml of water in and out of the stomach under gravity until a clear washing is obtained. (Usually × 4 is sufficient).
• Keep the initial aspiration sample for toxicology.
• Review the patient after 30 minutes or so following the procedure to exclude oesophageal perforation (subcutaneous emphysema clinically or by chest X-ray).

Contraindications
Ingestion of petroleum/kerosene/corrosive products.

Complications
Aspiration of gastric contents.

2. Forced diuresis

Indications
— Forced alkaline diuresis:
  ○ Plasma [salicylate] > 500 mg/litre.
  ○ Plasma [phenobarbitone] > 100 mg/litre.
  ○ Plasma [barbitone] > 100 mg/litre.
  ○ 2, 4-dichlorophenoxyacetic acid (2, 4-D).
— Forced acid diuresis:
  ○ Amphetamine.
  ○ Quinine (controversial).
  ○ Fenfluramine.
  ○ Phencyclidine.

The rationale behind the technique depends on the degree of ionization of the drugs involved as described in the Henderson–Hasselbach equation:

$$pH = pK_a + \log \frac{[HCO_3^-]}{[CO_2]}$$

When a drug is maximally ionized its lipid solubility is decreased, therefore an alkaline environment for weak acidic drugs and an acid environment for alkaline drugs will aid excretion.

Procedure
• Measure:
  ○ Arterial blood gases and pH.
  ○ Urea and electrolytes.
  ○ Blood sugar.
  ○ Urine pH.
• Insert central venous pressure line and urinary catheter and correct any pre-existing fluid depletion with appropriate fluid depending on plasma electrolytes.
• Proceed as follows:
  ○ forced alkaline diuresis:
     500 ml 5% dextrose ⎫
     500 ml 1.4% HCO₃ ⎬ hourly.
     500 ml 5% dextrose ⎭
  ○ forced acid diuresis:
     1 litre 5% dextrose ⎫
     500 ml 0.9% NaCl ⎬ hourly.
     10 g arginine HCl over 30 ⎬
     minutes ⎭

Continue in this manner rotating as necessary to maintain:
— Urine output $\geqslant$ 500 ml/hour (frusemide intravenously if necessary).
— For forced alkaline diuresis maintain urinary pH 7.5–8.5 by adjusting amount of HCO_3^- without increasing plasma pH above 7.6.
— For forced acid diuresis maintain urinary pH 5.5–6.5 by giving arginine as above or ammonium chloride 4 g every 2 hours.

K^+ should be added to the intravenous fluid as appropriate to keep $[K^+]$ in the normal range (usually 10–20 mmol/litre).

A reasonable approach (particularly if an on site flame photometer is available) is to measure:

Plasma electrolytes — 2-hourly.

Plasma pH — 2-hourly.

Urinary pH — hourly.

Urinary electrolytes — hourly (to assess electrolyte replacement).

Contraindications
— Significant pre-existing renal impairment.
— Pre-existing heart failure.
— Septicaemic shock.

Complications
— Fluid overload:
    ○ Pulmonary oedema.
    ○ Cerebral oedema.
— Gross osmotic swings—cardiovascular and acid-base instability.

7 Haematology

Data

1. Coagulation disturbances

The normal ranges shown in the table on page 136 are dependent on the methods used and the particular laboratory should be consulted.

2. Sickling disorders

- Screen all patients of Negroid and Arabian descent.
- Record the type of Hb in the notes.
- Consult with the haematology department before administering any anaesthetic or performing any operative procedure, unless sickle-cell trait HbAS.

3. Problems with large blood transfusions

- Febrile reactions:
  - Pyrogens in the apparatus.
  - White cell incompatibility.
  - Platelets and plasma protein reactions to recipient antibodies.
  - Allergic/anaphylactic reactions.
  - Transmission of disease from donor–recipient (e.g. malaria).
- Air embolism/microaggregate embolism.
- Hypothermia.
- Citrate toxicity.
- Hyperkalaemia.
- Acidosis.

Coagulation disturbances

	Platelet count (× 10^9/litre)	Prothrombin time (seconds)	Kaolin cephalin time difference (seconds)	Thrombin time (seconds)	Fibrinogen concentration (g/litre)	Fibrinogen degradation products (μg/ml)
Normal	200–400	Control = 10–14 seconds ± 2 seconds	Control = 28–33 seconds ± 7 seconds	Control = 10–12 seconds ± 2 seconds	1.4–3.0	< 10
Disseminated intravascular coagulation (DIC)*	↓	↑	↑	↑	↓	↑
Heparin	Normal	↑	↑	↑	Normal	Normal
Warfarin	Normal	↑	↑	Normal	Normal	Normal
Transfusion	↓	↑	↑	Normal	Normal	Normal
Impaired liver function	↓	↑	↑	Normal	Normal/↓	Normal/↑

* In DIC a fibrinogen level < 1.0 g/litre and a platelet count < 100 × 10^9/litre is diagnostic.

- Coagulation abnormality:
  - ↓ platelets.
  - ↓ factor V, VIII, XI.
  - Precipitation of DIC.
  - Functional platelet defect.
- Red cell incompatibility:
  - Haemolysis.
  - Acute renal failure.
-

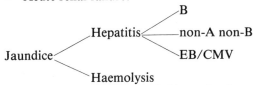

- Heart failure secondary to fluid overload.
- Acquired immune deficiency syndrome (AIDS).

Techniques

Bone marrow aspiration

Introduction

There are two types of samples obtainable, an aspirate and a trephine. Possible sites in the adult include the sternum (not suitable for trephine), posterior superior iliac spine (PSIS), anterior superior iliac spine (ASIS) and the vertebral processes. The ASIS approach will be described; this approach allows both trephine and aspiration biopsy and is of minimal concern to the patient.

Indications

Bone marrow biopsy is of use in a wide variety of haematological conditions, but it is also helpful in the investigation of many acute medical conditions (e.g. investigation of pyrexia of unknown origin—PUO).

Aspiration biopsy is of particular importance in suspected:
— Megaloblastic anaemia.
— Leukaemia.
— Sideroblastic anaemia.
— Thrombocytopenia.

Trephine biopsy, however, should be performed when the following seem likely:
— Aplasia.

— Myelofibrosis.
— Carcinomatous infiltration.
— Lymphoma (e.g. Hodgkin's disease).

Equipment
— Trolley.
— Dressing pack.
— Two aspiration needles (Salah).
— One Jamshidi trephine needle and probe.
— Gauze.
— 1% lignocaine.
— Two 20 ml syringes, one 10 ml syringe.
— No. 21 and 25G needles.
— No. 15 blade.
— Ten clean glass slides.
— One Pasteur pipette.
— One watch glass.
— One bicycle torch.
— Two sequestrene bottles.
— Collection bottles for culture, chromosomal analysis, etc.
— One stopwatch.

Procedure – aspiration biopsy
• Inform the patient of the intended procedure.
• Ensure the patient is not a haemophiliac and that the iliac crests have not previously been irradiated.
• Lie patient supine close to the right-hand side of the bed.
• Skin 'prep' and towel around the ASIS on the right having washed your hands thoroughly. Gloves are not necessary except in immunosuppressed patients.
• Identify the point of insertion which should lie 2 cm below the tip of the ASIS and 1 cm caudally.
• Infiltrate with 1% lignocaine (plain) down to the periosteum using No. 25 and 21G needles in succession in a fan-like manner and wait 2 full minutes (a stop watch is invaluable).
• Make a small incision in the skin with the No. 15 blade.
• Examine the Salah needle and remove the guard. Check that the stilette fits correctly and locks properly. Warn the patient that pressure but no pain will be felt over the site, and insert the needle through the skin at right angles to the iliac crest until the cortex is reached.
• Assuming the operator is right-handed (if not, the same

procedure on the left ASIS is easier) place the left index finger on the tip of the crest as a landmark and advance the needle in a twisting motion with pronation/supination of the wrist, first clockwise and then anticlockwise (as if holding a 'screwdriver'), until a 'give' is felt as the marrow cavity is entered.

It is not necessary to push very hard. In old and osteoporotic patients particularly, the entire iliac crest can be penetrated by overzealous attempts.

- Remove the stilette, attach a 20 ml syringe to the needle, warn the patient that they will feel a 'dragging sensation' in the hip and often in the right leg, and aspirate until a few millilitres of marrow enters the syringe.
- Place the entire contents in a sequesterene bottle and shake and reinsert the stilette. Send specimens of aspirate for culture, chromosomal analysis and electron microscopy if indicated.
- Pour some of the contents of the sequesterene bottle onto a watch glass and remove excess blood with a Pasteur pipette. If particles of marrow are visible, spread several slides and remove the Salah needle (a bicycle torch held under the watch glass is helpful for visualization of particles).
- If aspiration is unsuccessful initially, turn the needle through 90° and aspirate again. If still unsuccessful, withdraw the needle slowly whilst still aspirating. Repeat the procedure at a slightly different site if the tap is dry and, if the second sampling attempt is fruitless, perform a trephine.

Procedure – trephine biopsy
- The first seven steps are as above.
- Examine the Jamshidi trephine needle and choose a 4 inch 8 gauge size. Ensure the stilette is locked in position.
- Insert the needle at right angles to the crest and twist with a pronation/supination action (as above) until the marrow cavity is entered. Aspirate at this stage, if marrow has not already been obtained, having first removed the stilette.
- Then advance the needle further until a satisfactory sample is felt to have entered the needle (a further 5 mm approximately).
- Withdraw slightly, advance again but at a slightly

different angle and twist the needle 360° clockwise and then anticlockwise to secure the biopsy.
- Remove the needle *carefully* with slow pronating-supinating movements and by inserting the probe (provided) through the distal end of the needle the marrow sample can be removed without damage.
- If no sample is obtained, repeat the procedure in a slightly different site.
- Place the sample in formalin and send to the laboratory for processing (histology and haematoxylin and eosin, Giemsa, Romanowsky and reticulin staining).

Contraindications
— Haemophilia—full factor replacement will be necessary prior to biopsy if essential.
— Previous irradiation to site of aspiration.

8 Infection

Data

1. Notification of infectious diseases

If a viral haemorrhagic fever is suspected or diagnosed (lassa, marburg, ebola and smallpox), the patient and all contacts should be isolated and the appropriate Environmental Medical Officer (usually the District Community Physician) should be informed immediately. Hospital admission should be prevented if it has not already occurred, and arrangements made to transfer the patient to an infectious diseases unit.

The following diseases are also notifiable:

Anthrax.
Cholera*.
Diphtheria*.
Dysentry (amoebic or bacillary)*.
Encephalitis (acute).
Food poisoning*.
Infective jaundice.
Leprosy (directly to the DHSS).
Leptospirosis.
Malaria (contracted in UK).
Measles.
Meningitis (acute)*.
Ophthalmia neonatorum.
Paratyphoid*.
Plague.
Polio (acute).
Rabies*.
Relapsing fever.
Scarlet fever.
Smallpox.
Tetanus.
Tuberculosis.
Typhoid*.
Typhus.
Whooping cough.
Yellow fever.

* The District Community Physician should be informed by telephone as soon as appropriate rather than by the Notification of Infectious Diseases forms.

2. Control of hepatitis B in the ICU

1. Screen all high risk individuals (for venepuncture technique *see* 7 below):
   — Male homosexuals.
   — Recipients of multiple transfusions/blood products.
   — Haemophiliacs.
   — Drug addicts.
   — Tattooed patients.
   — Medical/paramedical staff as patients.
   — Jaundiced patients.
   — Prisoners/ex-prisoners.
   — Patients who have been dialysed.
   — Foreign patients.
   — Patients with chronic hepatitis.
2. Segregate (but do not necessarily isolate) HBsAg + ve patients who are bleeding, in danger of bleeding, incontinent or undergoing surgical treatment.
3. Reduce all blood contamination to a minimum ('Sharps' disposal box for needles, formal 'hepatitis risk' labelling for all specimens, 'double-bagging' of contaminated material).
4. Wear plastic aprons and gloves when handling spills or blood-contaminated linen, dressings, secretions and excreta.
5. Use sodium hypochlorite (ESH) or glutaraldehyde (Cidex) for all spillages.
6. Report all accidents (e.g. contaminated abrasions, needle-stick injuries, blood splashes into eye) to the Virology/Staff Health department for further advice concerning prophylactic use of immunoglobulin.
7. Perform a venepuncture as follows.
   — Write out request forms and leave outside room. Label specimen tubes.
   — Enter room with a polythene bag containing:
     ○ Pre-labelled specimen tubes with a Biohazard sticker or equivalent and appropriate laboratory bags.
     ○ Syringe/needle/sterile cotton wool balls.
     ○ Skin preparation (which should remain in the room).
     ○ Disposable gloves.
     ○ Disposable container.

- Place the polythene bag on a suitable surface and use it as a working area.
- Open the laboratory bags ready for the specimen tubes.
- Put on gloves, perform the venepuncture and fill the tubes.
- Place needle, syringe and cotton wool in the disposal container.
- Place the specimen tubes into their laboratory bags avoiding contamination of the outside of the tubes.
- Remove gloves and place them with the disposable container in the polythene bag.
- Leave the room, label the polythene bag and dispose of it in the waste room.

Control of acquired immune deficiency syndrome (AIDS) in the ICU

The acquired immune deficiency syndrome is described according to the Center for Disease Control (CDC) 1987 case-definition. It is divided into four groups.

CDC Classification of HIV disease

Group I   Acute infection.
Group II   Asymptomatic infection.
Group III Persistent generalized lymphadenopathy.
Group IV   Other diseases:
   Subgroup A — Constitutional disease.
   Subgroup B — Neurological disease.
   Subgroup C — Secondary infectious diseases.
      Cat C1 — Specified secondary infectious diseases listed in CDC definition of AIDS.
      Cat C2 — Other specified secondary infectious diseases.
   Subgroup D — Secondary cancers.
   Subgroup E — Other conditions.
The following individuals are at risk:
- Homosexual/bisexual men.
- Haemophiliacs.
- Intravenous drug abusers.
- Blood transfusion recipients.
- Female sexual partners of men at risk.

— Children of affected mothers.
— Caribbean connection (principally Haitian).
— Central African connection.

If AIDS is suspected:

1. Segregate (but do not necessarily isolate) patients who are bleeding, in danger of bleeding, incontinent or undergoing surgical treatment.
2. Prevent immunocompromised staff and pregnant staff (because the patient may excrete high levels of cytomegalovirus) from nursing the patient.
3. Reduce all blood contamination to a minimum ('sharps' disposal box for needles, formal Biohazard labelling for all specimens, 'double-bagging' of contaminated material).
4. Wear plastic aprons, gloves and goggles when handling spills or blood-contaminated linen, dressings, secretions and excreta.
5. Use freshly activated 2% glutaraldehyde, 2% phenolic disinfectant or freshly prepared 1% sodium hypochlorite for all spillages. If possible the disinfectant should be left in contact with the spillage for 30 minutes or so.
6. Report all accidents (e.g. contaminated abrasions, needle-stick injuries, blood splashes into the eye) to the Virology/Staff Health department for further advice.
7. Perform a venepuncture, with the added protection of goggles, having first alerted the appropriate laboratory of your intention, as described on page 142.

Drugs, dosages and infusion regimens

Antibacterial drugs

1. Amikacin

Use

Broad-spectrum aminoglycoside used in the treatment of Gram-negative infections resistant to gentamicin and/or tobramycin

Dosage

Intramuscular/intravenous bolus/infusion over 30 minutes 15 mg/kg per day in two divided doses (2.5 mg/ml).

NB
— Monitor plasma levels. Peak = 15–30 μg/ml. Trough
  $\leqslant$ 5–10 μg/ml.
— Consider pretreatment audiogram.
— Reduce dosage in renal impairment.
— Avoid concurrent administration of other
  ototoxic/nephrotoxic drugs.

2.   Amoxycillin

Use
Broad-spectrum penicillin used in the treatment of certain
Gram-positive and Gram-negative infections particularly:
* *Haemophilus influenzae.*
* *Escherichia coli.*
  It is inactivated by penicillinases.

Dosage
Oral
   250 mg 8-hourly.
Intravenous bolus/infusion
   500 mg–1 g 6-hourly.
NB
Hypersensitivity.

3.   Ampicillin

Use
Broad-spectrum penicillin used in the treatment of certain
Gram-positive and Gram-negative infections particularly:
* *Haemophilus influenzae.*
* *Escherichia coli.*
  It is inactivated by penicillinases.

Dosage
Oral
   250 mg 6-hourly.
Intravenous bolus/infusion
   500 mg 6-hourly.
NB
Hypersensitivity.

4.   Augmentin

Use
Penicillinase-producing bacteria resistant to amoxycillin.

Dosage
Oral
   375 mg 8-hourly.
Intravenous bolus/infusion
   1.2 g 8-hourly.
NB
—   Hypersensitivity.
—   Use with caution in hepatic impairment.
—   Reduce dosage in renal impairment.

5.   Azlocillin

Use
Broad-spectrum penicillin (a derivative of ampicillin) with
particular activity against *Pseudomonas aeruginosa*.

Dosage
Intravenous bolus
   2 g 8-hourly.
Intravenous infusion
   5 g 8-hourly.
NB
—   Hypersensitivity.
—   Reduce dosage in renal impairment to 12-hourly.

6.   Benzylpenicillin

Uses
Treatment of infections with:
*   *Streptococcus pyogenes* and *Streptococcus pneumoniae*.
*   *Streptococcus faecalis*.
*   *Neisseria gonorrhoeae* and *Neisseria meningitidis*.
*   *Haemophilus influenzae* (penicillin-sensitive).
*   Actinomyces.
*   *Bacillus anthracis*.
*   *Clostridium tetani*.
*   *Treponema pallidum*.
*   *Bacteroides* species and anaerobes.

Dosage
Intravenous bolus/infusion
  Up to 24 g/day in divided doses of 6-hourly.
NB
— Hypersensitivity.
— Convulsions with high doses.

7. Cefotaxime

Use
Broad-spectrum bactericidal cephalosporin similar to
cefuroxime but more potent against Gram-negative
organisms and *Pseudomonas*, and less potent against
Staphylococcus aureus.

Dosage
Intravenous bolus
  1 g 12-hourly.
Intravenous infusion
  1 g in 50 ml water for injection over 30 minutes 12-hourly.
NB
— Cross sensitivity with penicillins.
— Reduce dosage in renal impairment.
— Use with caution in combination with aminoglycosides
  or loop diuretics because of potential increased
  nephrotoxicity.

8. Cefuroxime

Use
Broad-spectrum bactericidal cephalosporin.

Dosage
Intravenous bolus/infusion
  750 mg–1 g 8-hourly.
NB
— Cross sensitivity with penicillins.
— Reduce dosage in renal impairment.
— Use with caution in combination with aminoglycosides
  or loop diuretics because of potential increased
  nephrotoxicity.
— Development of a positive Coomb's test in
  approximately 5% of patients interferes with blood
  cross matching.

9.   Ceftazidime

Use

Broad-spectrum bactericidal cephalosporin, active against a
wide range of Gram-positive, Gram-negative bacteria and
anaerobes.

Dosage

Intramuscular/intravenous bolus/intravenous infusion over
30 minutes

   1.0–6.0 g/day in two or three divided doses.

NB

— Cross sensitivity with penicillins.
— Reduce dosage in renal impairment.
— Use with caution in combination with aminoglycosides
   or loop diuretics because of potential increased
   nephrotoxicity.
— Development of a positive Coomb's test in
   approximately 5% of patients interferes with blood
   cross matching.

10.   Chloramphenicol

Use

Treatment of life-threatening infections with *Haemophilus
influenzae* when alternative therapy is inappropriate or
'blindly' in conjunction with pencillin in pyogenic
meningitis.

Dosage

Intravenous bolus/infusion

   50–100 mg/kg per day in four divided doses.

NB

Perform regular blood counts in view of the risk of
leucopenia, thrombocytopenia and irreversible aplastic
anaemia.

11.   Ciprofloxacin

Use

Broad-spectrum bactericidal fluoroquinolone particularly
active against Gram-negative bacteria which are resistant to
other antibiotics, including aminoglycosides, pencillins and
cephalosporins.

Dosage
Oral
  100–750 mg 12-hourly.
Intravenous infusion
  100–200 mg 12-hourly.
NB
— Reduce dosage in renal impairment.
— Theophylline is potentiated.

12. Co-trimoxazole

Uses
• *Pneumocystis carinii* pneumonitis.
• Nocardia pneumonitis.

Dosage
Oral
  8 adult tablets (480 mg each) 12-hourly for 14–21 days.
Intravenous infusion
  40 ml of intravenous solution (480 mg in 5 ml) diluted in 1
  litre of normal saline infused over 3 hours 12-hourly.
NB
— Use with caution in patients with hepatic impairment.
— Reduce dosage in renal impairment.

13. Erythromycin

Uses
• *Mycoplasma pneumoniae.*
• *Legionella pneumophilia.*
• Chlamydia.
• *Coxiella burneti.*
• As an alternative to penicillin in hypersensitive patients.

Dosage
Oral
  250–500 mg 6-hourly.
Intravenous bolus/infusion
  25–50 mg/kg per day in four divided doses.
NB
— Use with caution in patients with hepatic impairment.
— Theophylline is potentiated.

14.   Flucloxacillin

Use
Treatment of infections with *Staphylococcus aureus*
(penicillin sensitive and resistant).

Dosage
Oral
   250–500 mg 6-hourly.
Intravenous bolus/infusion
   250–500 mg 6-hourly.
NB
Hypersensitivity.

15.   Fusidic acid

Use
Treatment of infections with flucloxacillin resistant
staphylococci.

Dosage
Oral
   500 mg 8-hourly.
Intravenous infusion
   500 mg (over 6 hours) 8-hourly.
NB
Use with caution in patients with hepatic impairment.

16.   Gentamicin

Use
Broad-spectrum aminoglycoside for the treatment of Gram-
negative infections.
   Often given in combination with a penicillin and/or
metronidazole.

Dosage
Intravenous bolus
   2.0–5.0 mg/kg per day in three divided doses.
NB
—   Monitor plasma levels.
—   Reduce dosage in renal impairment.
—   Avoid concurrent administration of other
     ototoxic/nephrotoxic drugs.

17.   Metronidazole

Use
Treatment of anaerobic and protozoal infections.

Dosage
Oral
   400 mg 8-hourly.
Intravenous infusion
   500 mg 8-hourly.

18.   Mezlocillin

Use
Broad-spectrum penicillin particularly used for the treatment of infections with:
• *Escherichia coli.*
• *Proteus* species.
• *Pseudomonas aeruginosa.*

Dosage
Intravenous bolus/infusion
   2.0–5.0 g 6-hourly.
NB
— Hypersensitivity.
— Reduce dosage in renal impairment.
— Synergistic action with aminoglycosides.

19.   Netilmicin

Use
Broad-spectrum aminoglycoside for the treatment of Gram-negative infections.
   Similar to gentamicin, though reputed to be less nephrotoxic and ototoxic.

Dosage
Intramuscular/intravenous bolus/infusion over 30 minutes
   4.0–7.5 mg/kg per day in three divided doses reducing to twice daily according to response.
NB
— Monitor plasma levels.
— Reduce dosage in renal impairment.
— Avoid concurrent use of other ototoxic/nephrotoxic drugs.

20.   Piperacillin

Use

Broad-spectrum penicillin which is more active than mezlocillin in the treatment of infection with *Pseudomonas aeruginosa*.

Dosage

Intramuscular/intravenous bolus/intravenous infusion over 30 minutes

100–300 mg/kg per day in three or four divided doses.

NB
— Hypersensitivity.
— Reduce dosage in renal impairment.

21.   Pivampicillin

Use

Broad-spectrum penicillin used in the treatment of certain Gram-positive and Gram-negative infections particularly:
• *Haemophilus influenzae*.
• *Escherichia coli*.

It is inactivated by penicillinases.

Dosage

500 mg 12-hourly.

NB

Hypersensitivity.

22.   Rifampicin (for infusion)

Uses
• Pulmonary tuberculosis in patients unable to tolerate oral therapy.
• Broad-spectrum activity for the treatment of infection with Gram-positive and Gram-negative organisms particularly *Legionella pneumophilia*.

Dosage

Intravenous infusion

Single daily dose of up to 20 mg/kg over 2–3 hours to a maximum of 600 mg/day.

NB
— Reduce dosage in hepatic impairment.

—   Adjust dosage of relevant concurrent therapy (e.g. anticoagulants) because of liver enzyme induction.

23.   Ticarcillin

Use

Broad-spectrum penicillin used particularly for the treatment of infection with:
* *Proteus* species.
* *Pseudomonas aeruginosa.*

Dosage

Intravenous bolus (3–5 minutes) or intravenous infusion (30 minutes) of 15–20 g/day in divided doses at 4–8-hourly intervals.

NB
—   Hypersensitivity.
—   Reduce dosage in renal impairment.
—   Synergistic action with aminoglycosides.

24.   Tobramycin

Use

Broad-spectrum aminoglycoside with a spectrum which is similar to that of gentamicin but more active against *Pseudomonas aeruginosa.*
   It is claimed to be less nephrotoxic than gentamicin.

Dosage

Intravenous bolus
   3–5 mg/kg per day in three divided doses.

NB
—   Monitor plasma levels.
—   Reduce dosage in renal impairment.
—   Avoid concurrent administration of other ototoxic/nephrotoxic drugs.

Antiviral drugs

Influenza and the herpes viruses are the most important.

1. Acyclovir

Uses **and dosage**
- Patients with herpes simplex infections (with normal or impaired immune reponses) and in recurrent shingles (with normal immune responses):

    5 mg/kg by intravenous infusion over 1 hour at 8-hourly intervals for 5–7 days.
    (250 mg of freeze dried salt reconstituted in 10 ml of water for injection added to at least 50 ml of infusion fluid, for example 0.9% NaCl).
- Patients with varicella zoster infection (with impaired immune response) and in herpes simplex encephalitis:

    10 mg/kg by intravenous infusion over 1 hour at 8-hourly intervals for 5 days.

NB
— Monitor renal function closely because rises in serum creatinine and urea have been reported during treatment.
— Reduce dosage in renal impairment.
— Probenecid potentiates acyclovir.
— Acyclovir potentiates zidovudine.

2. Amantadine

Uses
- Herpes zoster.
- Prophylaxis in influenzae A contacts.

Dosage
100 mg p.o. twice daily for 14 days (herpes zoster) and 7–10 days for prophylaxis of influenzae A.
NB
— Reduce dosage in renal impairment.
— Epilepsy or a history of gastric ulceration are contraindications.

3. Idoxuridine

Uses
Topical treatment of herpes zoster and herpes simplex lesions of skin, external genitalia and eyes.

Dosage
Apply 5% solution to lesions 6-hourly. Use 40% in herpes zoster and apply 0.1% to eyes.

4.   Vidarabine

Uses
- Herpes simplex I and II.
- Herpes zoster and vaccinia.
- Cytomegalovirus (CMV).

Dosage
Ophthalmic ointment
  3% 5 times/day for 7 days at least.
Parenteral solution
  10 mg/kg per day for at least 5 days.
NB
— Reduce dosage in renal impairment.
— Bone marrow suppression occurs occasionally.

5.   Foscarnet (clinical trial/named patient basis)

Uses
- Herpes viruses.
- Cytomegalovirus (CMV).
- Human immunodeficiency virus (HIV).

Dosage
24 mg/ml solution should be administered via a central line. For peripheral vein administration dilute to 12 mg/ml by piggy-backing with an equal volume of 5% dextrose/ dextrose saline or normal saline. Dosage is calculated according to serum creatinine and body weight.
NB
— Reduce dosage in renal impairment.
— The incidence of nephrotoxicity and hypocalcaemia is increased if pentamidine is given concurrently.

6.   Ganciclovir (clinical trial/named patient basis)

Use
Cytomegalovirus (CMV).

Dosage
Intravenous infusion
   5 mg/kg over 1 hour for 10–20 days.
Maintenance
   3 mg/kg b.d. or 5 mg/kg daily for 5–7 days (add required
   dose of 250 mg in 5 ml solution to 100–250 ml of 5%
   dextrose/normal saline).
NB
— Reduce dosage in renal impairment.
— Bone marrow suppression is dose related.
— Myalgia occurs occasionally.

7.   Zidovudine

Use
Human immunodeficiency virus (HIV) in patients with
AIDS or ARC (AIDS-related complex).

Dosage
Oral
   3.5 mg/kg 4-hourly. Reduce to 8-hourly if Hb < 9g/dl or
   neutrophil count < 1.0×10^9/litre. Stop if Hb < 7g/dl
   or neutrophil count < 0.75×10^9/litre.
   Review after two weeks and recommence at a dose every
   8 hours if appropriate.
   NB
— Bone marrow toxicity is frequent and serious (*see*
   above).
— Reduce dosage in renal and hepatic impairment.
— Nausea, headache, myalgia, insomnia, seizures and a
   polymyositis syndrome have been described.

Antifungal drugs

1. Imidazoles	2. Polyenes	3. Synthetic
clotrimazole	amphotericin B	flucytosine
miconazole	nystatin	
econazole	natamycin	
isoconazole	candicidin	
ketoconazole		
ticonazole		

Specific use and dosage

(*a*) *Oral/oesophageal candidiasis*
— Attend to dentures.
— Drug treatment:
   ○ Amphotericin lozenges/suspension — 1 lozenge/1 ml suspension four times daily for 14 days.
   ○ Nystatin suspension — 100 000 units 6-hourly continued for 48 hours after the lesions have resolved.

(*b*) *Systemic infections*
   Candidiasis.
   Cryptococcal meningitis.
   Fungal endocarditis.
   Rhinocerebral mucormycosis.
   Blastomycosis, coccidioidomycosis, histoplasmosis, paracoccidioidomycosis.
   Pulmonary/cerebral aspergillosis.

— Drug treatment
   ○ Slow intravenous infusion of amphotericin in 5% dextrose over 6 hours.
      — 250 μg/kg increasing to a maximum of 1.5 mg/kg in severely ill patients. (A 50 mg vial is dissolved in 10 ml of water for injection to give a 5 mg/ml solution. The required dose is then added to 5% dextrose to give a concentration of no more than 0.1 mg/ml. The resulting solution is stable for 8 hours and should be protected from light.)

NB
— The high dose schedule can be given on alternate days as amphotericin is excreted slowly.
— Reduce dosage in renal impairment.
— Hypokalaemia, hypomagnesaemia and bone marrow depression have all been reported.
   ○ Intravenous flucytosine.
      150–200 mg/kg in four divided doses, each over 20–40 minutes.
— Avoid monotherapy if possible as resistance may develop.

— Bone marrow suppression (especially involving white blood cells).
  ○ Intravenous amphotericin and flucytosine (synergistic action).
  ○ Miconazole
    Intravenous infusion over 30 minutes of 600 mg (3 ampoules) 8-hourly. Dilute in 200–500 ml of 5% dextrose/normal saline.
— Care in patients with cardiovascular disorders.
— Potentiation of anticoagulants, antiepileptic and hypoglycaemic drugs.

Antiprotozoal drugs

Pentamidine isethionate

Use
Pneumonia due to *Pneumocystis carinii*.

Dosage
4 mg/kg daily for at least 14 days.
Intramuscular
  300 mg dissolved in 3 ml of water for injection deep into the buttock.
Intravenous infusion
  300 mg dissolved in 3–5 ml of water for injection and then diluted further in 50–250 ml of 5% dextrose/normal saline. Infuse over at least 60 min. in the supine position.
Inhalation
  600 mg dissolved in 6 ml of water for injection. Inhale via a nebulizer with a flow rate of 6–10 litres/min. for 21 days.
NB
— Perform baseline FBC, blood sugar, LFTs, urea and creatinine.
— Reduce dosage in renal impairment.
— Beware hypotension following i.m. or rapid i.v. injection.
— Hypo- and hyperglycaemia may occur.
— Bone marrow suppression described.

Index